# THE CLUBFOOT

# THE CLUBFOOT

## WALLACE B. LEHMAN, M.D.

*Physician-in-Charge*
*Pediatric Orthopedic Surgery*
*Soroka Medical Center*
*Ben Gurion University of the Negev*
*Beersheva, Israel*

*Medical Director and Chief Pediatric Orthopedic Surgery*
*Children's Orthopedic Hospital of Jerusalem*
*Jerusalem, Israel*

## With a contribution by GABRIEL TOROK, M.D.

*Professor of Orthopedic Surgery*
*Director of the Department of Orthopedic Surgery*
*Soroka Medical Center*
*Ben Gurion University of the Negev*
*Beersheva, Israel*

*Illustrated by*
*Hugh Thomas*
*Medical Illustrator*

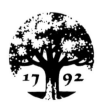

## J. B. LIPPINCOTT COMPANY
*Philadelphia*       Toronto

*Printed in the United States of America*
    2   4   6   8   9   7   5   3   1

**Library of Congress Cataloging in Publication Data**

Lehman, Wallace B
    The clubfoot.

    Includes index.
    1.  Clubfoot — Surgery.  I.  Torok, Gabriel, joint author.  II.  Title. [DNLM:  1.  Club-foot — Surgery. WE883 L523c]
RD783.L38              617'.398              79-22402
ISBN 0-397-50457-8

לאבי ואמי

גבריאל וועלוול בן שמואל חיים ודאבע ציביע

באר־שבע, תשל״ט

*To all those people—*
*relatives, teachers,*
*colleagues, patients—*
*upon whose shoulders*
*I have stood to*
*produce this guide*

# INTRODUCTION

I am a physician doomed to the Practise of Surgery.
                                                    Lord Moynihan

What comes from a single pen here in the desert of the Negev concerning the clubfoot is small in relation to what has come already from pens throughout the world, yet I believe that my experience will be a useful contribution to the field of clubfoot treatment. I make no excuse for what is contained in the following pages, but neither do I expect my conclusions to go unquestioned.

There is no doubt in my mind that there are many paths to the satisfactory correction of clubfoot, and I would have been delighted to include here discussions of the benefits and disadvantages, as I see them, of all the various procedures, but this was impossible. I therefore take full responsibility for the results of my choices, and I ask understanding of those people whose work I have failed to mention. If I come to see that I have omitted something important, I hope I will learn from this and continue to work toward the goal of lessening the number of badly treated clubfeet. But now, this book represents what I feel to be the method of treatment which will lead to the greatest number of useful feet.

Because I so strongly stress the need for early surgical treatment of the clubfoot, I think it fitting to also remind my readers of the words of John Hunter:

> This last part of Surgery, namely operations, is a reflection on the healing art. It is tacit acknowledgment of the insufficiency of Surgery. It is like an armed savage who attempts to get that by force which a civilised man would get by stratagem. No surgeon should approach the victim of his operation without a sacred dread and reluctance. (Quoted by Sir Reginald Watson-Jones, February 16, 1959, in his Hunterian Oration to the Royal College of Surgeons.)

# ACKNOWLEDGMENTS

A book is never truly a one-man job, but it would be impossible for me to adequately acknowledge the many people who contributed, directly or indirectly, to this book. However, some individuals deserve special thanks. The late Dr. Daniel Casten, the teacher who first interested me in becoming a surgeon, is one. He was the first surgeon to show me what hard work, study, and respect for the patient and for my colleagues was all about. All I know about surgery came from him.

Of the other teachers at the Hospital for Joint Diseases who nurtured me, I must thank especially Dr. Bernard Kleiger, who first encouraged my interest in the clubfoot and to whom I frequently refer in the following pages; Dr. Joseph Milgram, past Director, who was able to show me how to empathize with the patient; and Dr. Herman Robbins, present Director, who has always been a friend and who imparted to me the importance of anatomy during those late nights studying with him and his stale sandwiches. I must thank those who taught me how to operate—Sidney Bernstein, Murray Burton, Mel Jahss, Leo Mayer, Mark Lazansky—and those who taught me how to think—Charles Sutro, Henry Mankin, Henry Jaffee, and Emanual Kaplan. And thank you, Dr. Alex Norman, for my knowledge of x-ray.

To my associates in New York, Dr. Ralph Hirschhorn, Dr. Harvey Orlin, and Dr. Steve Borkow, who gave me the encouragement and the time to write and in whose office I gathered most of my experience with the clubfoot, and especially to Dr. Hirschhorn for being my friend—thank you.

To my wonderful dedicated secretaries, Alice Altmeyer at the Hospital for Joint Diseases, my dear Tanya Shevins at the Long Island Orthopaedic Group, and Bilha Savell at the Ben Gurion University of the Negev—thank you for putting up with me and deciphering my handwriting. To the entire staff of the Long Island Orthopaedic Group, thank you.

Many thanks to the Director of Orthopaedic Surgery at the Soroka Medical Center in Beersheva and to Professor Gabriel Torok who not only encouraged me but made the book better with his marvelous chapter on the neglected clubfoot. Thanks to the entire staff of Ben Gurion—the photographer, Annate, and all those who aided me. And thanks to Professor Moshe Prywes for being the guiding light for Ben Gurion where I was able to write this book; I am grateful for my time in Israel where so much of what we know about the clubfoot has originated.

To Hugh Thomas whose exceptional illustrations for this book make it not only useful but beautiful, thank you.

To the people of Lippincott, especially Stuart Freeman and Lisa Biello, I owe my thanks for their organizational expertise and for keeping me going.

And to my wife and children, Margorie, Nancy, and Danny. How can I repay the time I've taken from them? Without their encouragement and their doing without a husband and father, this book would never have been completed. I promise to give them all my time from now on—until the next book.

# CONTENTS

# THE CLUBFOOT

# 1 WHAT IS A CLUBFOOT?

Before we consider the treatment of the clubfoot (talipes equinovarus), it is necessary to understand the terminology which is currently used to describe it. The term *talipes equinovarus* is derived from the Latin: *talipes*, a combination of the words *talus* (ankle) and *pes* (foot); *equinus*, meaning "horselike" (the heel in plantar flexion); and *varus*, meaning inverted and adducted.

The deformity is one of the more common congenital deformities, occurring in 1 to 2 per 1,000 live births.

There are many other varieties of the clubfoot, such as valgus (everted heel) and calcaneus (dorsiflexion of the heel), (Fig. 1–1). Almost any combination of these varieties may be seen. This monograph, however, will be dealing with the most common variety—talipes equinovarus, which is usually referred to as the clubfoot (Figs. 1–2, 1–3, 1–4).

At birth the diagnosis can be made by observing the foot for the three basic deformities (Fig. 1–5):

1. *Forefoot adduction.*
2. *Hindfoot inversion, usually associated with supination and called varus. For simplicity I will refer to this as hindfoot inversion.*
3. *Hindfoot equinus.*

I believe there is also a fourth basic deformity of the true clubfoot, a medial subluxation of the navicular on the head of the talus (Kleiger, 1962). This is not easy to see or demonstrate clinically at birth, but after some experience it can easily be felt.

*1*

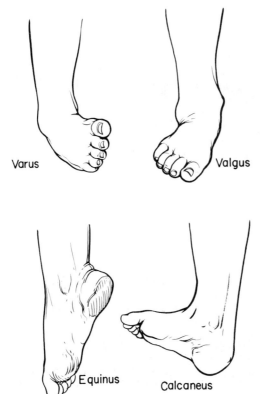

Varus          Valgus

Equinus          Calcaneus

Fig. 1–1. Primary deformities of the foot and ankle.

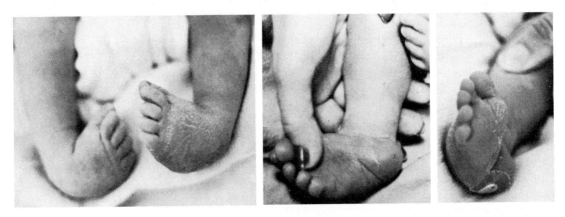

Fig. 1–2A. *(Left)* Infant with clubfoot, view from the front: inversion of foot
and inversion of heel. Fig. 1–2B. *(Middle)* Infant with clubfoot, medial view:
inversion of heel, hindfoot equinus (nurse holding adductus in slight correction). Fig. 1–2C. *(Right)* Infant with clubfoot, view from front with leg in
slight external rotation: inversion of heel, forefoot adductus, equinus heel,
varus of foot.

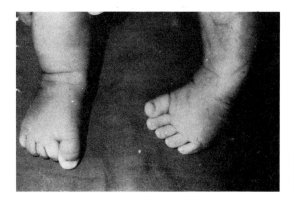

Fig. 1–3A. Four-month-old with unilateral club-foot, view with both feet on floor: adductus of foot, inversion of foot.

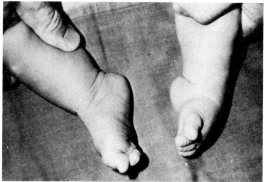

Fig. 1–3B. Four-month-old with unilateral club-foot, medial view of feet: adductus of foot, inversion of heel, and equinus of heel.

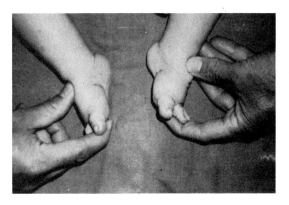

Fig. 1–3C. Four-month-old with unilateral club-foot, medial view with attempt to correct equinus: equinus of heel fixed, adductus and inversion of foot.

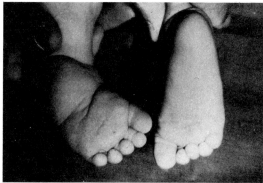

Fig. 1–3D. Four-month-old with unilateral club-foot, view of sole of foot: adductus of foot, inversion of heel, and small heel (bean-shaped).

A great majority of normal children have at birth what may appear to be a clubfoot, but in reality is simply an intrauterine positional attitude which will correct itself in a few days or weeks. It has always been my habit to mentally classify all children with possible clubfoot deformities into two basic categories:

Type I—Nonrigid: those which correct easily and may simply be a persistent intrauterine position

Type II—Rigid: those which are difficult to correct manually or are very severe deformities (Attenborough, 1972)

It is essential that the above distinction be made. The variation in results between reporters (Kite, 1930, 1964) who claim 80 to 90 percent good results in

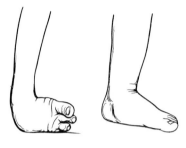

Fig. 1–4. Adolescent with clubfoot, neglected, unilateral. All elements can be seen: forefoot adductus, inversion of heel, inversion of foot, equinus heel. (After kite, The Clubfoot. New York, London, Grune & Stratton, 1964.)

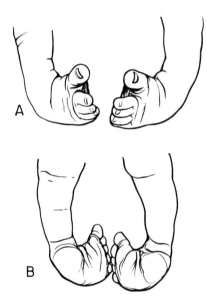

Fig. 1–5. Newborn clubfoot. A. Frontal view: forefoot adductus; inversion of forefoot, and inversion of heel. B. View from the rear: inversion of heel, forefoot adductus, equinus of heel. (After Kite, The Clubfoot. New York, London, Grune & Stratton, 1964.)

nonoperative treatment and those who claim only 30 to 50 percent good results in nonoperative treatment (Lloyd-Roberts, 1971; and Wynne-Davis, 1964) may simply be related to the type of clubfoot being treated. When the deformities are separated into Types I and II, it is possible to achieve 100 percent positive results with the Type I deformities, whether plaster or manipulation is used, and close to 0 percent good results in Type II using nonoperative treatment. I think that in a clubfoot which is manually easily correctable, with a soft springy feel in a relatively normal sized foot, one should be able to obtain close to universal success nonoperatively. With small feet, rigid with atrophic muscles (bean-shaped foot) (Lloyd-Roberts, 1971), which I consider Type II, I anticipate at best a 50 percent success rate nonsurgically, but probably closer to 30 percent. Fifty to 70 percent of such deformities will require some type of operative correction.

Before proceeding to the treatment of the clubfoot we must be sure that we are dealing with a congenital clubfoot and there are no associated condi-

**Table 1–1.** *Classification of Clubfoot*

| *Classification related to type of treatment expected* | |
|---|---|
| I. Nonrigid type | Probably related to intrauterine position (Packing syndrome) |
| II. Rigid type | True clubfoot with all basic elements |
| III. Resistant rigid type | Clubfoot seen in association with other diseases, such as arthrogryposis and myelomeningocele, or in association with other congenital deformities (tetralogical clubfoot) |

tions which will compromise our treatment. The child with a myelomeningo-cele, a tibial deficiency, arthrogryposis, or other congenital anomalies will certainly present additional problems in management. Treatment of the clubfoot itself in children with arthrogryposis or meningomyelocele is much more difficult and resistant for not only conservative treatment, but operative treatment as well. In fact, a third category of deformities, Type III, should include those children with arthrogryposis or meningomyelocele (See Table 1–1). No surgeon who has treated the clubfoot of an arthrogrypotic child would consider such a case the same as an ordinary clubfoot. They are much more difficult to treat and much more resistant to treatment. In fact, there are possibly some who should not be treated because treatment is a losing battle.

Before discussing the anatomy and pathoanatomy of the clubfoot, a brief word about etiology is in order. Much has been written about the etiology of the congenital clubfoot, but its exact cause has not been determined and can only be speculated upon. The list of incriminating causes is endless but may be broken down into basic categories (Table 1–2). Both Hippocrates (400 B.C.) and Galen (200 A. D.) considered the clubfoot to be caused by extrinsic pressure of the fetus in utero (Kite, 1964). Many writers up to the present day still consider this one cause, if not the only cause (Wynne-Davies, 1964). Of course, the hereditary germ plasm theory must be considered, and there is no doubt that clubfoot deformities occur much more frequently in those families that already have a member with a clubfoot (Palmer, 1964).

A marvelous study of the evolution of the normal foot and the clubfoot was done by Böhm in 1929. He was able to show that the variation we see in

**Table 1–2.** *Etiology of Clubfoot*

1. Extrinsic pressure of embryo in utero
2. Nerve lesion
3. Hereditary – germ plasm deficiency
4. Arrested embryonal development
5. Bone anomalies
6. Failure of muscle development
7. Congenital dislocation of the navicular or talus
8. Circulatory – temporary or permanent breakdown of circulation

clubfoot relates to physiological positions that can be seen in the normal embryonal development of the foot — very convincing evidence of the embryonal
arrest theory.

Irani and Sherman (1963) and others, especially Settle (1963), have meticu-
lously dissected abnormal and normal feet and found various bony, muscular,
and circulatory abnormalities which led them to believe that primary distur-
bances in bone are the cause of the clubfoot. In my own experience in the operating room, these abnormalities have been quite evident. I remember one of
my most respected teachers pointing out to me at the operating table "the dislocated navicular and the menicus of soft tissue" (Kleiger, 1962). Are what we
see in surgery the cause of the congenital clubfoot, or is the clubfoot caused by
such factors as primary nerve lesion causing muscle imbalance, as in meningomyelocele, primary muscle disease causing unbalanced pull on the foot (Handelsman, 1965), or impairment of circulation causing fibrosis of tissues and
contractures? Is the clubfoot caused by a combination of the above factors? Or
is it caused by none of these factors, but simply the result of a dislocation of
the navicular on the talus? Kite's quote from Ecclesiastes (200 B.C.) is most
apt: "Thou knowest not . . . how the bones do grow in the womb of her that is
with child."

Finally, let us consider what clubfoot is and is not, radiologically. The use
of x-rays in the assessment of clubfoot is twofold. First, x-rays both in the an-
teroposterior (A-P) or superior-inferior view and in the lateral view of the foot
are used preoperatively in my clinic to assess the severity of the clubfoot. I
might add here that clinically the surgeon's judgment is much more important
preoperatively than x-ray evaluation. Second, x-rays are used in the operating
room postoperatively (Turco, 1971; Ashby, 1973) and intraoperatively (Simons, 1978) to determine the degree of correction obtained; here it is most
important *not* to use clinical judgment but to rely on the x-ray. Before the skin
is closed, an appropriate x-ray will demonstrate whether the proper structures
have been released. The relapsed clubfoot seen frequently in the past is most
likely the result of not taking x-rays of a postoperative clinically normal foot
in which the talocalcaneal joint was not corrected.

The x-ray technique that we use has been recommended by Beatson and
Pearson (1966) and reemphasized by Turco (1971) and Ashby (1973). It should
be remembered when reading the x-rays that the primary centers of ossification of the talus, calcaneus and cuboid are visible in the infant. However, the
ossification center of the navicular may not appear until age 3 years. The
metatarsals and phalanges are all present on x-ray at birth. Two views are
taken; the A-P view, sometimes called the superior-inferior view, with the
foot in 30 degrees of plantar flexion (Beatson and Pearson, 1966), and the lateral view, which I take with the foot at a right angle to the ankle and which
Beatson recommends to take also with the foot in 30 degrees of flexion.

On these x-rays lines are drawn to measure angles. On the A-P view two
lines are drawn, one through the center of the longitudinal axis of the talus

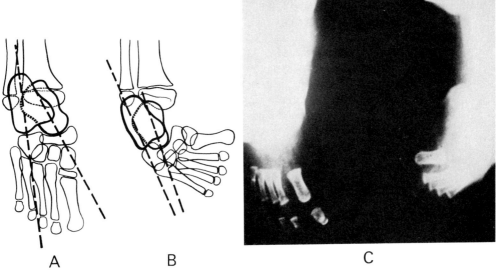

Fig. 1–6A & B. X-ray A-P view, with two lines drawn, one along the longitudinal axis of the talus, and one through the center of longitudinal axis of the calcaneus. A. Diagram of A-P x-ray of normal foot. B. Diagram of A-P x-ray of severe clubfoot. C. Actual x-ray of child shown in Fig. 1–3 with left clubfoot.

parallel to its medial border and one through the longitudinal axis of the calcaneus parallel to its lateral border. In the normal foot the line through the talus will point to the first metatarsal and the line through the calcaneus will point to the cuboid or fifth metatarsal, thus forming a "V." This angle should measure 20 to 40 degrees. The more severe the clubfoot, the more closely the lines approach being parallel, indicating that the calcaneus is lying under the talus or is inverted. In a severe clubfoot the lines may both point to the fifth metatarsal or laterally, indicating overlapping of the talus and calcaneus (Fig. 1–6).

As correction proceeds, the calcaneus rotates out of inversion and the angle moves toward 40 degrees. This angle is called the talocalcaneal angle or Kite's angle. In the lateral view, two lines are again drawn—one line through the longitudinal axis of the talus parallel to its inferior border and the second through the longitudinal axis of the calcaneus parallel to its inferior border. This talocalcaneal angle should measure between 35 and 50 degrees. In the clubfoot the angle approaches 0 degrees and may even be minus a few degrees. In other words the more severe the clubfoot the closer to parallel the lines become (Fig. 1–7).

Postoperatively we place most emphasis on the lateral view in the operating room. The lateral view is taken with the foot in slight dorsiflexion; if the calcaneus and talus are no longer parallel, the talocalcaneal joint has been freed. Therefore, the lateral x-ray is an invaluable guide in the operating room.

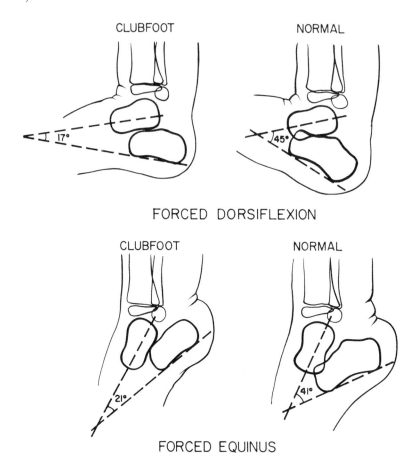

CLUBFOOT                    NORMAL

17°                         45°

FORCED DORSIFLEXION

CLUBFOOT                    NORMAL

21°                         41°

FORCED EQUINUS

Fig. 1–7. Diagrams of lateral x-rays of normal foot and clubfoot in forced dorsiflexion and forced equinus. Lines are drawn through the longitudinal axis of the talus parallel to the inferior border of the talus and through the longitudinal axis of the calcaneus parallel to the inferior border of the calcaneus.

Unless this view shows restoration of the normal angle of the talocalcaneal joint, the operation is not finished. X-rays may also be used in evaluating other stages of the clubfoot, such as the "rocker-bottom" foot in which the line of the calcaneus that would ordinarily pass through the calcaneocuboid joint passes below the joint. Also, if a deformed "flat-topped talus" is seen on x-ray, you can be sure forced manipulation preoperatively or postoperatively has been done and osteochondral compression of the cartilage has occurred. The probable result of cartilage compression caused by persistent forceful manipulation of the clubfoot or inadequate surgical release would be a degenerative, painful osteoarthritic foot—a good reason for doing nothing to the clubfoot either with manipulations or surgery, since osteoarthritis and pain are not seen in the neglected untreated clubfoot (Herold and Torok, 1973).

Simons (1978) has taken the radiological treatment of the clubfoot even further. In what he calls the "analytical" or "progressive" approach to the treatment of the clubfoot he preoperatively catalogues the variations of deformity using x-rays. During surgery x-rays are used stage by stage to determine exactly what releases are necessary to obtain correction of the clubfoot. This is a most interesting approach to the treatment of the clubfoot, and it is exactly this type of thinking that I have tried to apply to my approach. The same surgical procedure cannot be done on every clubfoot, therefore during surgery it is necessary to evaluate each step to decide what needs to be done to correct *that particular* clubfoot.

# REFERENCES

Ashby, M.: Roentgenographic assessment of soft tissue medial release operations in clubfoot deformity. Clinical Orthop. 90:146–149, 1973.

Attenborough, C. G.: Early posterior soft tissue release in severe congenital talipes. Equinovarus. Clinical Orthop. 84:71, 1972.

Beatson, T. R. and Pearson, J. R.: A method of assessing correction in clubfoot. J. B. & Jt. Surg. 48:40, 1966.

Böhm, M.: The embryological origin of the clubfoot. J. B. & Jt. Surg. 11:229, 1929.

Garceau, G. J.: Talipes equinovarus. American Academy of Orthopedic Surgeons Instructional Course Lectures, Vol. 7, Ann Arbor, J. W. Edwards, 1950.

Handelsman, J. E., Youngleson, J. and Malkin, C.: A modified approach to the Dwyer os calcis osteotomy in clubfoot. S. Afr. Med. J. 39:989, 1965.

Herold, H. Z, and Torok, G.: Surgical correction of neglected clubfoot in the older child and adult. J. B. & Jt. Surg. 55-A: 1385, 1973.

Irani, R. N. and Sherman, M. S.: The pathological anatomy of the clubfoot. J. B. & Jt. Surg. 45-A: 45, 1963.

Kite, J. H.: Non-operative treatment of congenital clubfoot. A review of one hundred cases. South. M. J. 23: 337–345, 1930.

Kite, J. H.: The Clubfoot. New York, London, Grune & Stratton, 1964.

Kleiger, B.: Significance of tibiotalar navicular complex in congenital clubfoot. J. Hosp. Joint Dis. 23:158, 1962.

Kleiger, B. and Mankin, H. J.: A roentgenographic study of the development of the calcaneus by means of the posterior tangential view. J. B. & Jt. Surg. 43-A: 961–969, 1961.

Lloyd-Roberts, G. C.: Orthopaedics in Infancy and Childhood. London, Butterworths, 1971.

Palmer, R. M.: The genetics of talipes equinovarus. J. B. & Jt. Surg. 46-A: 542, 1964.

Settle, G. W.: The Anatomy of Congenital Talipes Equinovarus. J. B. & Jt. Surg. 45-A:1341, 1963.

Simons, G.: Analytical radiography and the progressive approach in talipes equinovarus. Orthopedic Clinics of N. A. 9, 1:187, 1978.

Turco, V. J.: Surgical correction of the resistant clubfoot: One-stage posteromedial release with internal fixation. A preliminary report. J. B. & Jt. Surg. 53: 477, 1971.

Wynne-Davies, R.: Family Studies in clubfoot. J. B. & Jt. Surg. 46-B: 445, 1964. Review of treatment of clubfeet. J. B. & Jt. Surg. 46-B: 464, 1964.

# 2  A BRIEF HISTORY OF THE CLUBFOOT

Since Hippocrates' time the clubfoot has remained a most difficult and perplexing problem for the orthopedic surgeon to treat successfully. It is Hippocrates who is given credit for the first known description of the clubfoot (Hippocrates, 1927). He recognized that early gentle manipulations with bandages could be surprisingly effective. In 1743 Nicholas Andry, in his "orthopaedia," described a deformity of the foot resembling the foot of a horse, which he called "Pedes Equinal" (Andry, 1743). It was not until 1831, when Stromeyer began using tendo-Achillis tenotomy, that surgery became part of the treatment of the clubfoot (Brockman, 1930). Little of London (1839), who underwent tendo-Achillis lengthening, continued this treatment with some success. Although even before Stromeyer, reports by Lorenz (1784), Sartorius (1812), and Delpech (1816) indicated that subcutaneous tenotomies were being done frequently for clubfoot (Kuhlmann, 1972).

The clubfoot is common enough to have been described in modern literature: Somerset Maugham in *Of Human Bondage*, Gustave Flaubert in *Madame Bovary* (Maugham, 1915; Flaubert, 1857).

The artistic world did not neglect the clubfoot. There are several sixteenth-century paintings depicting the clubfoot, such as "Madonna and Child" by Lucas the elder, and "The Clubfoot" by José Ribera (Ruhräh, 1932, 1933).

There has been no limit to the ingenious devices that have been used to correct the clubfoot, mostly remnants of medieval torture devices. One such instrument used in the sixteenth century to correct a clubfoot in a prince involved turnscrews (Bohne, 1938). I, myself, discovered in the basement of the Hospital for Joint Diseases a Thomas wrench which had been used to forcefully manipulate a clubfoot — it was a large wrench which encased the forefoot or heel (Telson, 1926). Forrester-Browne, as recently as 1936, used a clamp to evert the heel in the early stages of treatment (Forrester-Browne 1936). It sounds primitive, but may not be much different from some of the manipulations I have done with plaster casts.

While in my early years as an orthopedic surgeon during the early 1950s, it was impressed upon me that treatment of the clubfoot produced a large percentage of poor results. I was taught to consider the treatment of the clubfoot in two stages: (1) before maturity one should try to obtain the best foot possible with manipulations, plaster casts and soft tissue surgery and (2) after maturity, accomplish a definitive correction with triple arthrodesis (Hanisch, 1953).

Since that time there have been many studies of the results of early manipulation of the clubfoot all leading to agreement that about 25 percent of all those treated for clubfoot end up with a poor result (Lloyd-Roberts, 1971; Shaw, 1964; Fripp and Shaw, 1967). It is interesting to note that Lloyd-Roberts (1971) in his analysis of the use of manipulation and Denis Browne splints not only found a 25 percent failure rate, but using Kite's method of plaster correction only corrected 2 out of 17 feet. His experience reflects mine and other's that the use of Kite's method can only successfully complete the treatment in approximately 30 to 70 percent of clubfoot cases.

Kite's plaster correction technique has been a great influence on everyone who treats the clubfoot. Today, either his technique or a similar technique, such as frequent strapping and manipulation, is used. I realized shortly after I began treating the clubfoot that Kite's results of nearly 90 percent correction could not be reproduced. I still believe in his technique and use it first on all children; however, at present I do not continue the technique if I feel it is not effective, and will consider other treatment after 2 to 4 months.

Supporting evidence for this has been given by Wynne-Davies (1964), who showed that she was only able to correct 30 percent of feet by plaster without operation. In 1930 Brockman also obtained only 50 percent correction with stretching and manipulation, but increased his results to 70 percent after using his posterior release. I can correct approximately 70 percent of the total clubfoot deformities nonsurgically — excluding the postural deformities which correct 100 percent of the time — and the rest need surgical correction. In the severe clubfoot with a small heel, my results go down to 30 to 40 percent successes nonoperatively. I believe I can feel clubfeet at birth and know which one will do well with plaster and which will need surgery.

There is at present a resurgence of enthusiasm for using soft tissue and hard tissue surgery early in the history of the disease to obtain as normal a foot as possible as early as possible, rather than using surgery as a salvage, such as in triple arthrodesis. This attempt is not new. In 1784 Lorenz tried tendo-Achillis tenotomy and Sartorius in 1812, but because of the high incidence of infection it was not until Lister's teaching of asepsis that even the subcutaneous tenotomies of Delpech in 1816 (Fergusson, 1843) and Stromeyer (Stromeyer, 1835) had some success.

The orthopedic surgeon by his very nature has not neglected using the surgical approach in attempting to correct the clubfoot. The poor little bean-shaped foot has received the benefits of the greatest surgeons' skill, but not always for the everlasting benefit of the foot. All clubfoot clinics are full of the relapsed or recurrent or shall we say "poorly treated" clubfoot. These feet usually have many scars and, in fact, are rigid with scar tissue from misdirected manipulations and surgery. I have been guilty of this myself and can produce my own cases of recurrent clubfoot. It is hoped that the enthusiasm I have today for the surgical correction of the recalcitrant and relapsed clubfoot will continue and not result in the disenchantment which has occurred in the past.

There has been much enthusiasm in the past for the tendo-Achillis tenotomy, soft tissue release (Brockman, 1930), posterior release (Attenborough, 1972), and radical soft tissue release (Bost, 1960); however, the initial enthusiasm waned and now has been reborn. We have all blamed poor postoperative care and inadequately performed surgery by inadequately prepared surgeons for the failure. Again early radical surgery is being advocated. What is different today? The answer to that could involve a book in itself, but let me try to analyze why I think we are on the threshold of being able to correct nearly all congenital clubfoot at an early age.

Why should surgery be carried out early? Everyone treating clubfoot deformities has experienced the foot resulting from multiple manipulations and surgical procedures which have not completely corrected the problem. The foot is rigid, deformed, not serviceable, and certainly not belonging to a happy patient. Can deformities be prevented from progressing by early surgery? There is no doubt that we as treating physicians are causing damage to growing epiphyseal centers and soft cartilaginous tissue by our forceful methods. The sooner we bring the tissues closer to the normal anatomy, the fewer deforming forces will persist. There is no justification, after a few well-intentioned manipulations have failed, for persisting and creating pressure defects on growing bone. It is possible today with sharp, meticulous, gentle soft-tissue dissection to bring the foot to almost normal anatomical relationships. Our present advanced knowledge of the anatomy of the talocalcaneo navicular joint complex will allow more accurate judgment of what elements of the clubfoot have to be released to obtain normal anatomical relationships. It is now possible at an early age (2 to 3 months) for the surgeon to realize which foot is not making progress and what has to be done to allow the foot to develop satisfactorily to skeletal maturity.

A further look into the following chapters of this text should enable the surgeon to understand surgically what the clubfoot is all about and what procedures are available to correct the deficiencies found. I hope it will also be realized by the surgeon that each foot is different and requires other procedures, either surgical or nonsurgical, and that at some point each foot may require variations of both the surgical and nonsurgical treatment.

The interested reader is directed to a complete review of the history of the treatment of the clubfoot deformity in Kite's *The Clubfoot* (1964). In this review Kite quotes E. H. Bradford: "The literature on the treatment of clubfeet is, as a general rule, that of unvarying success. It is often as brilliant as an advertising sheet and yet in practice, there is no lack of half-cured or relapsed cases, sufficient evidence that methods of cure are not universally understood" (Bradford, 1889).

# REFERENCES

Andry, N.: Orthopaedia (facsimile reproduction of the first edition in English, London, 1743). Philadelphia, J. B. Lippincott, 1:212–224.

Attenborough, C. G.: Early posterior soft tissue release in severe congenital talipes Equinovarus. Clinical Orthop. 84:71, 1972.

Bohne, O.: Orthopedic treatment of clubfoot in the 16th Century. Z Krüppel Fürsorge 31:104, July–August, 1938.

Bost, F. C., Schottstaedt, E. R. and Larsen, L. J.: Plantar dissection. An operation to release the soft tissues in recurrent or recalcitrant talipes equinovarus. J. B. & Jt. Surg. 42:151, 1960.

Bradford, E. H.: Treatment of clubfoot. Trans. Am. Orthopedic A. 1:89–115, 1889.

Brockman, E. P.: Congenital Clubfoot. New York, Wood, 1930.

Fergusson, W. A.: Delpech Cited in a System of Practical Surgery. Philadelphia, Lea and Blanchard, 1843, p. 350.

Forrester-Browne: A clamp for stretching congenital clubfoot. Lancet 1:897, 1936.

Flaubert, G.: Madame Bovary, 1857. New York, Bantam Books, 1959.

Fripp, A. T. and Shaw, N. R.: Clubfoot. Edinburgh, Livingstone, 1967.

Hanisch, C.: Director of Clubfoot Clinic, Hospital for Joint Diseases. 1958.

Hippocrates. Loeb Classical Library (Trans. Dr. E. T. Withington) vol. 3. London, Heinemann, New York, Putnam, 1927.

Kite, J. H.: The clubfoot. New York, London, Grune & Stratton, 1964.

Kuhlmann, R.: A survey and clinical evaluation of the operative treatment for congenital talipes equinovarus. Clinical Orthop. 84:88, 1972.

Lister, J.: On a new method of treating compound fractures, abscess, etc. with observations on the conditions of suppuration. London, Lancet, Part 1: 364; Part II, 2: 418, 622, 1867.

Little, W. J.: A Treatise on Clubfoot. London, 1839.

*17*

Lloyd-Roberts, G. C.: Orthopaedics in Infancy and Childhood. London, Butterworths, 1971.

Lorenz, A.: Ueber Die Operative Orthopedie des Klumpfusses, Wien, Urban and Schwanzenberg, 1889, form Hft. 5 & 6 of Wien Klinik, p. 117.

Maugham, S. W.: Of Human Bondage, New York, Doubleday, 1915.

Ruhräh, J.: Pediatrics in Art, congenital deformity. Am. J. Dis. Child. 43:714, 1932.

Ruhräh, J.: Pediatrics in Art, clubfoot. Am. J. Dis. Child. 46:1397, 1933.

Sartorius, J. F.: Gluckliche Herstellung eines verkrummten Fusses durch die Durchschneidung der Achillessehne. In von Siebold Annstadt, J. B. (ed.): Sammlung Seitner und auserlesener chirugischer Beobach tungen and Erfahrungen, Vol. 3, 1812, p. 258.

Shaw, N. E.: Clubfoot comparison of three methods of treatment. Br. Med. J. 1: 1084, 1964.

Stromeyer, L.: Cited in Division of the tendo-Achillis in clubfoot. Lancet 2: 648, 1835–36.

Telson, D.: A clubfoot wrench. J. B. & Jt. Surg. 8:425–426, 1926.

Wynne-Davies, R.: Family Studies in clubfoot. J. B. & Jt. Surg. 46-B: 445, 1964. Review of treatment of clubfeet. J. B. & Jt. Surg. 46-B: 464, 1964.

# 3 ANATOMY

The understanding of the talocalcaneonavicular joint complex is essential for the treatment of the clubfoot. Without intimate knowledge of the anatomy of this joint in its normal and pathological states, the surgeon's ability to treat the clubfoot is precluded. The joint is complicated and in some ways difficult to visualize simply through words and pictures. I would recommend to all surgeons who attempt clubfoot surgery to go back to the dissecting laboratory at least a few times to examine the anatomy which I will be describing in this chapter. There is much written about and much controversy over the etiology of the clubfoot, but there is general agreement concerning the normal anatomy of the talocalcaneonavicular joint and the pathological anatomy we find at surgery. The anatomy is basic, must be understood, and can be understood with a little time and dissection.

Let us first consider the entire talocalcaneonavicular (TCN) joint complex and its various parts and ligaments. Table 3–1 demonstrates all those ligaments which will be of interest to us in performing an adequate clubfoot operation. The joints we are concerned with are the ankle joint, the subtalar joints both anterior (talocalcaneonavicular) and posterior (talocalcaneal), and the midtarsal joint including the calcaneocuboid joint.

The TCN joint is a ball and socket joint — the ball being the head of the talus and the socket formed laterally by the bifurcated ligament (the Y ligament of the subtalar joint), anteriorly by the navicular, and dorsomedially by the deltoid ligament, talonavicular ligament and posterior tibial tendon (Figs. 3–1, 3–2, and 3–3). The floor of the ball and socket joint is formed by the middle and anterior articular surfaces of the calcaneus and the strong calcaneo-

**Table 3–1.**  *Ligaments to Be Dealt with in Surgery of the Clubfoot*

A. *Talocalcaneonavicular Joint Complex*
  1. Subtalar joint—articulation between the talus and calcaneus, consists of 2 articulations
    a. Anterior joint—the talocalcaneonavicular joint, consisting of 3 ligaments
      (1) dorsal talonavicular
      (2) interosseous talocalcaneal ligament
      (3) plantar calcaneonavicular ligament (spring ligament)
    b. Posterior joint—talocalcaneal joint
      (1) anterior talocalcaneal ligament
      (2) posterior talocalcaneal ligament
      (3) lateral talocalcaneal ligament
      (4) medial talocalcaneal ligament
      (5) interosseous talocalcaneal ligament

  2. Midtarsal joint—also called transverse tarsal joint (Gardner, 1975), consisting of the talonavicular joint and the calcaneocuboid joint
    a. Talonavicular joint—that part of the midtarsal joint described above as the anterior part of the subtalar joint
    b. Calcaneocuboid joint
      (1) dorsal calcaneocuboid ligament
      (2) bifurcated ligament (Y ligament)
      (3) long plantar ligament
      (4) plantar calcaneocuboid ligament

B. *Ankle Joint*
  1. Medial aspect of the ankle joint
    a. "Master knot of Henry"
    b. Deltoid ligament—medial ligament of the ankle joint
      (1) deep
      (2) superficial
        (a) anterior tibionavicular
        (b) middle calcaneotibial
        (c) posterior talotibial

  2. Posterior aspect of the ankle joint
    a. Lateral ligament of the ankle joint
      (1) calcaneofibular ligament
      (2) talofibular—posterior portion
    b. Posterior-inferior tibiofibular ligament—crural interosseous ligament (Both posterior-inferior tibiofibular ligament and crural interosseous ligament are known as ligaments of the syndesmosis of the ankle joint.)
    c. Posterior capsule of subtalar joint
    d. Posterior capsule of ankle joint

  3. Lateral aspect of the ankle joint (The only ligament to concern us here is the calcaneofibular portion of the lateral ligament of the ankle joint.)

navicular (spring ligament). The navicular, cuboid and calcaneus all seem to move together because of strong ligamentous attachments. Movements all occur around the ball of the socket, the talus, and in the subtalar and midtarsal joints (see Fig. 3–1).

Let us first consider the posterior aspect of the ankle and subtalar joints. Posteriorly we must be able to see:

> 1. *Posterior inferior tibiofibular ligament extending from the posterolateral aspect of the tibia distally to the post aspect of the fibula, covering over the interosseous ligament of the ankle joint*

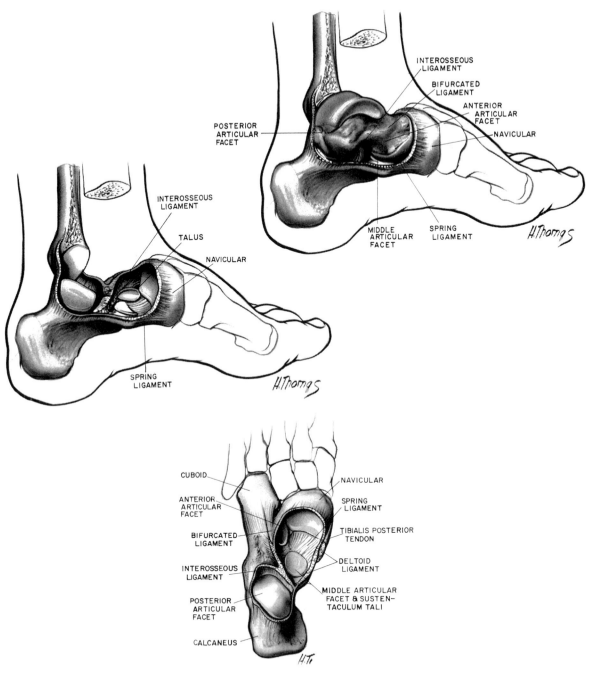

Fig. 3-1. *(Top)* Medial view of the talocalcaneonavicular joint with medial malleolus, distal tibia and deltoid ligament removed.

Fig. 3-2. *(Middle)* View of talocalcaneonavicular joint with talus removed. This joint is a ball and socket joint: the ball is the head of the talus and the socket formed laterally by the bifurcated ligament, anteriorly by the navicular, and dorsomedially by the deltoid ligament, talonavicular ligament, and tibialis posterior tendon. Note the strong interosseous ligament.

Fig. 3-3. *(Bottom)* View of the floor of the talocalcaneonavicular joint.

21

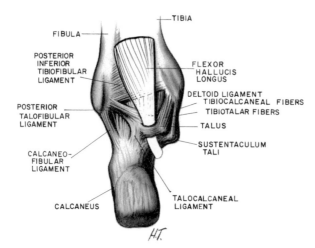

FIBULA

TIBIA

POSTERIOR INFERIOR TIBIOFIBULAR LIGAMENT

FLEXOR HALLUCIS LONGUS

DELTOID LIGAMENT
TIBIOCALCANEAL FIBERS
TIBIOTALAR FIBERS

POSTERIOR TALOFIBULAR LIGAMENT

TALUS

SUSTENTACULUM TALI

CALCANEO-FIBULAR LIGAMENT

TALOCALCANEAL LIGAMENT

CALCANEUS

H.T.

Fig. 3–4. Posterior aspect of the ankle joint. We see the posterior inferior tibiofibular ligament (below which is the interosseous ligament of the ankle joint), deltoid ligament, posterior talofibular ligament, talocalcaneal ligament, and calcaneofibular ligament. The flexor hallucis longus tendon is in the way of the posterior joint capsule.

2. *Calcaneofibular ligament—that portion of the lateral ligament of the ankle joint extending from the fibula to the lateral aspect of the calcaneus*

3. *Deltoid ligament—posterior portion only of the superficial deltoid ligament*

4. *Posterior portion of the talofibular ligament—in reality a thickened part of the posterior capsule of the ankle joint extending from the talus and probably also from the tibia to the posterior medial portion of the fibula*

5. *Talocalcaneal ligament of the posterior subtalar joint—we should be able to see the posterior, medial, and lateral portions of the talocalcaneal ligament*

6. *Interosseous ligament of the subtalar joint—after the subtalar joint is opened we should be able to see the thickened veil of the interosseous ligament. Of course, the tendon of the flexor hallucis longus would be in the way posteriorly (Fig. 3–4).*

Medially we should see (Fig. 3–5A, B, C):

1. *"Master knot of Henry." A very thick, heavy structure made up of fibrous tissue and cartilage which extends from the navicular around the flexor digitorum longus and flexor hallucis longus tendons to reattach to the navicular or the fascia of the flexor hallucis brevis. The knot is sometimes included in a large mass of scar tissue and cartilage which is partly attached to the navicular and medial malleolus and may be the primary tissue holding the navicular in its displaced position (Kleiger, 1962).*

2. *Deltoid ligament—only its superficial anterior, middle, and posterior portions attached to the calcaneus. The deep portion of the deltoid ligament attached to the talus from the inner aspect of the medial malleolus of the tibia is only visualized after the superficial deltoid ligament is removed (see Fig. 3–8).*

3. *Navicular—usually displaced medially*

4. *Talus—usually found lateral to the medially displaced navicular*

5. *Plantar calcaneonavicular ligament—extending from the sustentaculum*

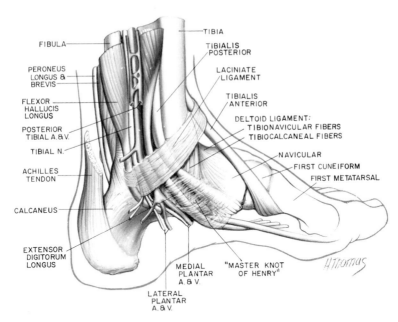

Fig. 3–5A. Medial aspect of ankle joint. The tendons: *Achilles tendon, posterior tibial tendon, tibialis anterior, flexor hallucis longus* and *flexor digitorum longus* including the *neurovascular bundle* (posterior tibial nerve and artery) are all superficial. Note the "Master knot of Henry."

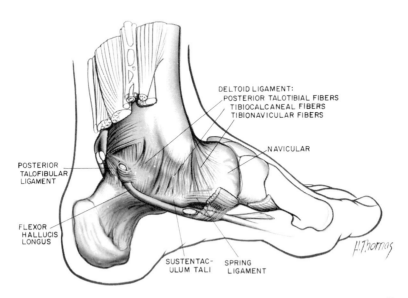

Fig. 3–5B. Medial aspect of ankle joint with tendons cut away, showing all the ligaments of the inner side of the joint.

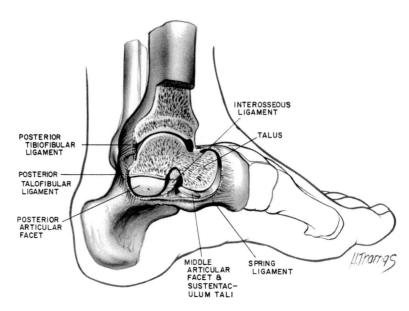

POSTERIOR
TIBIOFIBULAR
LIGAMENT

POSTERIOR
TALOFIBULAR
LIGAMENT

POSTERIOR
ARTICULAR
FACET

INTEROSSEOUS
LIGAMENT

TALUS

MIDDLE
ARTICULAR
FACET &
SUSTENTAC-
ULUM TALI

SPRING
LIGAMENT

Fig. 3–5C. Medial aspect of ankle joint with part of medial malleolus and talus cut away showing the interosseous ligament.

*tali of the calcaneus to the medial border of the navicular (spring ligament)*

6. *Medial talocalcaneal ligament of the subtalar joint only seen after the deltoid ligament is sectioned*

7. *Talonavicular ligament — medial and dorsal portions*

8. *Neurovascular bundle — the deltoid ligaments and underlying structures are all covered by the posterior tibial tendon, posterior tibial nerve artery, and vein, flexor digitorum longus and the flexor hallucis longus*

After sectioning the deltoid ligament and medial subtalar ligaments (the talocalcaneal ligaments) we should see:

1. *Long plantar ligament — extending from the calcaneus to the cuboid*

2. *Bifurcated ligament — extending from the calcaneus to the cuboid and lateral aspect of the navicular*

3. *Interosseous ligament of the subtalar joint which is probably just a thickening of the anterior capsule of the posterior subtalar joint and a thickening of the posterior capsule of the anterior subtalar joint (Fig. 3–6)*

If all the above anatomy is seen by the operating surgeon and he is familiar with this anatomy, proceeding on to the actual surgery of the clubfoot should not be difficult.

To further clear up any misunderstanding of the function of the subtalar and ankle joints, a brief discussion of the movements occurring in dorsiflexion and plantar flexion of the foot is in order. In plantar flexion and dorsiflexion of the foot, motion occurs both in the tibial-talar joint (ankle joint) and in the talocalcaneonavicular joint (subtalar joint). This is a complex combined motion and I will not go into its biomechanics at this time. Let us simply say that pure dorsiflexion and plantar flexion occurs at the ankle joint, however, combined with this motion is a rotation of the calcaneus around the talus. Actually the rotation (inversion and eversion of the calcaneus) occurs around the talus with the calcaneus, cuboid, and navicular acting as one unit because of their strong ligamentous attachments — probably the interosseous membrane of the subtalar joint acting as a pivot. In dorsiflexion the foot comes up and the heel goes into eversion, and the foot assumes a position of pronation. The anterior portion of the calcaneus moves laterally with the navicular and cuboid, and the posterior portion of the calcaneus moves downward. In plantar flexion of the foot the calcaneus inverts; the navicular cuboid and calcaneus all move as one unit, rotating under the talus. The foot assumes an attitude of supination and equinus (normal equinovarus attitude). The anterior end of the calcaneus moves downward and medially while the posterior end moves upward and laterally. Templeton (1965) showed radiographically that varus and valgus movement occurs at the middle and anterior subtalar articulations. Very little motion occurs in the talonavicular joint and at the calcaneocuboid and posterior subtalar articulations.

Much has been written about the causes of the pathomechanics and pathoanatomy of the talocalcaneonavicular joint, and much has been written about why we see what we see at surgery; however, most is speculation. There are two points which I think have been proven: (1) there is a deformity of the talus — a medial deviation and downward deviation of the neck of the talus — which is consistently found in the resistant clubfoot but not always in the nonrigid clubfoot (Waisbrod, 1973; Settle, 1963; Irani and Sherman, 1963); (2) in all clubfoot surgery, we can consistently see an inversion of the calcaneus and a medial displacement of the navicular, indicating some type of dislocation or subluxation of the navicular-cuboid-calcaneus complex around the talus (Turco, 1971; Settle, 1963). To these two points there can be very little disagreement (Fig. 3–7).

If we consider the congenital clubfoot as a fixed exaggeration of the normal equinovarus position and as a dislocation of the navicular-cuboid-calcaneus complex on the talus, we can expect to see certain contractures medially, posteriorly and in the subtalar joint. It is these contractures that prevent us from obtaining a reduction of the foot in the resistant clubfoot.

The contractures that we find surgically as a rule are:

1. *Medially:*
   a. *Posterior tibial tendon, the flexor hallucis longus tendon, and the flexor digitorum longus tendon are all shortened, occasionally also the abductor hallucis longus.*
   b. *The navicular is displaced medially and fixed in scar tissue usually, in some cases against the tibia.*
   c. *Deltoid ligament*

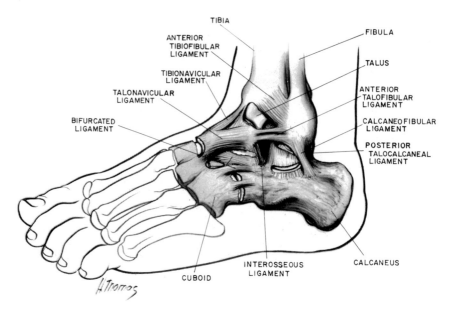

Fig. 3–6. Lateral aspect of the joint. The interosseous ligament can be seen laterally.

    *d. Talonavicular joint capsule*
    *e. Spring ligament (the plantar calcaneonavicular ligament)*
    *f. Plantar fascia contracture*

*2. Subtalar contractures:*
    *a. Bifurcated ligament*
    *b. Interosseus ligament*

*3. Posteriorly:*
    *a. The talus may be almost subluxed forward out of the mortise of the*
       *ankle joint with an inability of the talus to fit back into the mortise —*
       *contracture of the distal tibiofibular syndesmoses*
    *b. Achilles tendon*
    *c. Talofibular ligament*
    *d. Calcaneofibular ligaments*

    Turco (1971) and others add that the Achilles tendon may also be attached medially on the calcaneus, adding to the deformity. It is possible that inversion of the heel only makes this seem to occur, but in any event releasing the Achilles tendon from its insertion medially on the calcaneus helps correct the deformity.

    It is most important to remember that, to be corrected, the subtalar complex must be released both anteriorly and posteriorly for the navicular-cuboid-calcaneus complex to move around the talus. It is the *fixed* navicular which prevents movement of the subtalar joint. In the uncorrected clubfoot, the posterior part of the calcaneus is up, fixed by the posterior contractures, and the

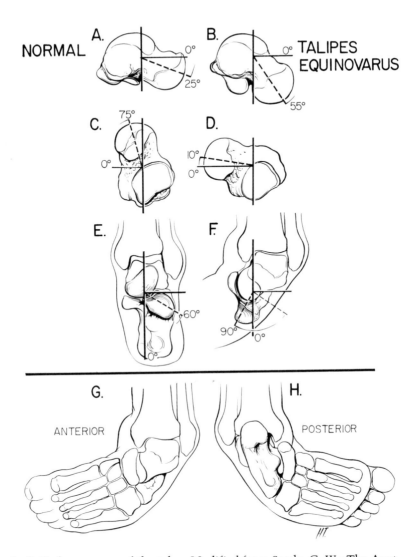

Fig. 3–7. Pathoanatomy of the talus. Modified from Settle, G. W.: The Anatomy of congenital talipes equinovarus. J.B. & Jt. Surg. 45-A: 1341, 1963. In the left-hand column A, C, and E are drawings of normal tali; in the right-hand column are the tali of congenital equinovarus. It can be seen that in equinovarus the neck of the talus is deviated downward and medially and is foreshortened. The calcaneus is also inverted under the talus, as can be seen in F as compared with E. The facet for the cuboid is rotated underneath the talus. The final deformity of the foot can be seen in G and H.

anterior part of the calcaneus is down, fixed by the medial contractures. If the calcaneus is released posteriorly, we cannot expect the anterior portion of the calcaneus to move upward and evert around the talus until it too is released. It is most important to remember that usually a posterior release, medial release, or subtalar release is not enough alone. All contractures have to be released in order to reduce the displaced navicular and calcaneus. There may be exceptions in that sometimes we see clubfeet which have contractures more pronounced posteriorally or medially, and therefore might not need extensive release, but these are less common.

It has been suggested by Brockman (1930) and Steindler (1920) that cavus is a part of the deformity and must be released as well. I do not see much cavus in the earlier age groups, but when I do I add a plantar fascia release to the operation. In the older child a cavus is very often present and sometimes will require bone surgery.

Let me add a word here about three controversial issues concerning the anatomy of the clubfoot. The first issue is the importance of the interosseous ligament of the subtalar joint. There are surgeons doing clubfoot surgery who do not feel it is a very important structure, and, in fact, some are not even certain it exists. However, the interosseous ligament does exist and is always found to be present if one looks for it. It may not be severely contracted in all cases; in fact, in many cases I have operated on, correction of the clubfoot has occurred before the interosseous ligament was encountered. I have also had several cases in which the surgical correction is a struggle until this very heavy, small contracted interosseous ligament is released. Though the ligament is always present, it varies in importance to the severity of the clubfoot. If the surgeon is having difficulty, release of this ligament may have surprising results (Fig. 3–8).

The second issue involves the deformity of the talus. I think there is no doubt about the medial deviation and downward inclination of the talus. I think there are also subluxations of the talus forward out of the ankle mortise. There is no question that it is occasionally necessary to release the distal tibiofibular joint, cutting the posterior inferior tibiofibular ligament and crural interosseous ligament so that the talus can be dorsiflexed back into the mortise (syndesmectomy). Why this is more common in England and seemd to be found more in the English literature than elsewhere I cannot say. However, the subluxation forward of the talus does occur and dorsiflexion of the talus may be impossible without releasing this syndesmosis. Maybe this is the "rotatory luxation of the talus" described by Burr Curtis (Curtis, 1978).

The third controversial point is the age-old controversy of internal and external tibial torsion. Wherever one reads about the clubfoot, tibial torsion is mentioned—internal tibial torsion by Brockman (1930), Kite (1964), and Salter (1970). I was taught that in spite of the literature external tibial torsion occurs in clubfoot deformity (Kleiger, 1962). This was also thought to be the case by Lloyd-Roberts (1974) and Swann (1969). In 1964, Wynne-Davies reported that she found no case of tibial torsion outside of the normal range. In 1976, Herold

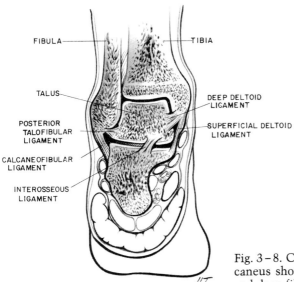

FIBULA

TIBIA

TALUS

DEEP DELTOID
LIGAMENT

POSTERIOR
TALOFIBULAR
LIGAMENT

SUPERFICIAL DELTOID
LIGAMENT

CALCANEOFIBULAR
LIGAMENT

INTEROSSEOUS
LIGAMENT

Fig. 3–8. Cross-section of the talus and calcaneus showing the interosseous ligament and deep fibers of the deltoid ligament.

and Marcovich, using three techniques of tibial measurement including the x-ray measurement of Rosen and Sandick (1955), also found no evidence of tibial torsion. I have been unable to demonstrate internal or external tibial torsion in any of the clubfeet that I have seen in patients below the age of 8. In the neglected clubfoot I have seen internal tibial torsion which I suspect is the response of the tibia during growth to the gait pattern of the clubfoot walk. In the neglected clubfoot in the older age group there may be a place for osteotomy of the tibia, but otherwise I think not.

# REFERENCES

Brockman, E. P.: Congenital Clubfoot. New York, Wood, 1930.

Curtis, B.: Sound Slide Program. Pediatric Orthopedic Conference of the American Academy of Orthopedic Surgeons, 1978.

Gardner, E., Gray, D. and O'Rahilly, R.: Textbook of Anatomy. Philadelphia, W. B. Saunders, 1975, p. 244.

Herold, H. Z. and Marcovich, C.: Tibial torsion in untreated congenital clubfoot. Acta Orthopedia Scand. 47: 112, 1976.

Irani, R. N. and Sherman, M. S.: The pathological anatomy of the clubfoot. J. B. & Jt. Surg. 45-A: 45, 1963.

Kite, J. H.: The Clubfoot. New York, London, Grune & Stratton, 1964.

Kleiger, B.: Significance of tibiotalar navicular complex in congenital clubfoot. J. Hosp. Joint Dis. 23:158, 1962.

Lloyd-Roberts, G. C.: Orthopaedics in Infancy and Childhood. London, Butterworths, 1971.

Lloyd-Roberts, G. C., Swann, M. and Caterall, A.: Medial rotation osteotomy for severe residual deformity in clubfoot. J. B. & Jt. Surg. 56-B: 37, 1974.

Rosen, H. and Sandick, H.: The measurement of tibiofibular torsion. J. B. & Jt. Surg. 37-A: 847, 1955.

Salter, R. B.: Textbook of Disorders and Injuries of the Musculoskeletal System. Williams & Wilkins, 1970, p. 93.

Settle, G. W.: The anatomy of congenital talipes equinovarus. J. B. & Jt. Surg. 45-A: 1341, 1963.

Steindler, A.: Stripping of the os calus. J. Orthopedic Surg. 2:8 – 12, 1920.

Swann, M., Lloyd-Roberts, G. C. and Caterall, A.: The anatomy of uncorrected clubfeet. A study of rotation deformity. J. B. & Jt. Surg. 51-B: 263 – 269, 1969.

Templeton, A. W., McAlister, W. H. and Zim, I. D.: Standardization of terminology and evaluation of osseous relationships in congenitally abnormal feet. Am. J. Roentgen-ol. 93:374, 1965.

Turco, V. J.: Surgical correction of the resistant clubfoot: One-stage posteromedial release with internal fixation. A preliminary report. J. B. & Jt. Surg. 53: 477, 1971.

Waisbrod, H.: Congenital clubfoot: An anatomical study. J. B. & Jt. Surg. 55-B: 796, 1973.

Wynne-Davies, R.: Family Studies in clubfoot. J. B. & Jt. Surg. 46-B: 445, 1964. Review of treatment of clubfeet. J. B. & Jt. Surg. 46-B: 464, 1964.

# 4 CONSERVATIVE TREATMENT OF THE CLUBFOOT

The purpose of this monograph is to explain the anatomy and pathoanatomy of the clubfoot and to arrange in some order the progressive treatment of the clubfoot, emphasizing the early use of surgery in those feet which are resistant to nonsurgical efforts. To be complete, I have included here a brief discussion of the nonsurgical treatment of the clubfoot which can be expected to correct at least 50 percent of clubfoot deformities or as many as 90 percent (Kite, 1964).

Basically there are at present two methods of nonoperative treatment: the manipulative and strapping method, used mostly in England and Europe, and the gentle plaster manipulative treatment popular in the United States.

Let me emphasize that the first attack on an untreated clubfoot, whether in the newborn or the older neglected child, should be nonsurgical. The nonsurgical treatment can be effective in two ways: (1) by completely correcting the clubfoot, as the definitive treatment; (2) by partially correcting a clubfoot, thereby making the surgical approach less extensive and possibly even converting what could have been a radical soft tissue release into simply a posterior release.

The question of how early the clubfoot should be treated and how late is too late is easily answered: it is never too early and never too late. All orthopedic surgeons have been brought up on the maxim, in a breech delivery the clubfoot cast should be on the foot before the head is delivered. I know of at least one overeager house officer who was found in the delivery room doing just that. The point to be made is that the earlier the treatment of the clubfoot is started, the easier the treatment is and the better the results. On the other

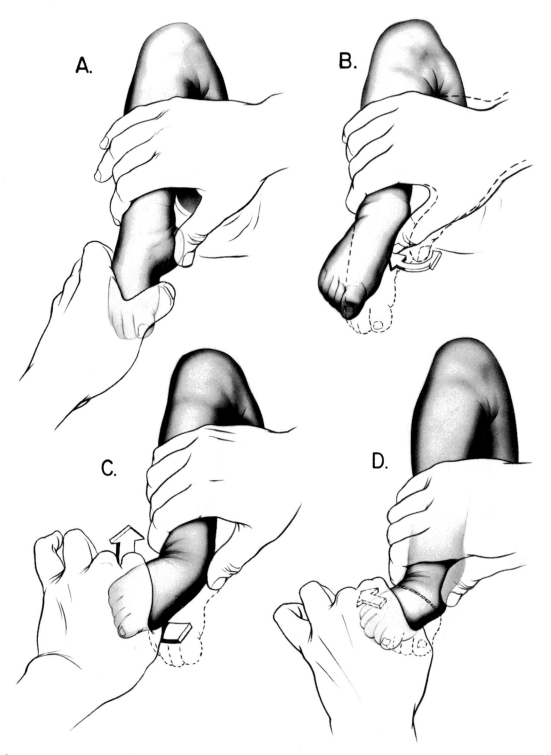

Fig. 4–1. Manipulation of foot. A. Left hand with thumb manipulates right forefoot; right thumb manipulates right heel. B. Right thumb manipulates right heel. C. Right thumb is relaxed. D. Left thumb and index finger manipulate forefoot into eversion and abduction.

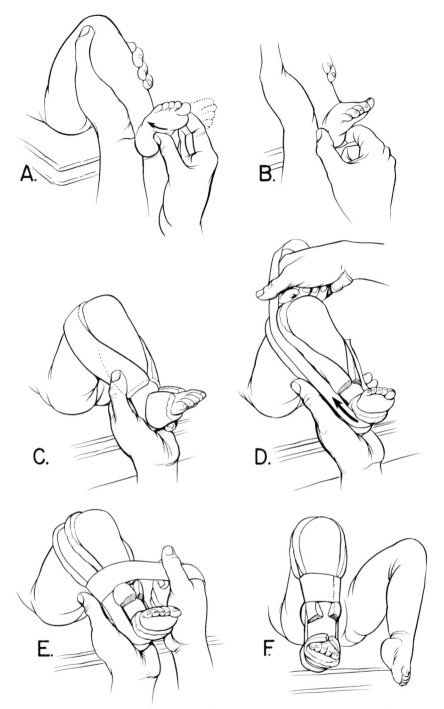

Fig. 4-2. Robert Jones strapping of the clubfoot. A. Gently, the surgeon manipulates the forefoot outward with thumb and index finger. B. The same is done with the heel, turning it into eversion. C. After two felt straps are applied as shown, D. tape is applied in two strips. The first tape is applied from the forefoot, medially, bringing the foot into abduction, and then up the outer side of the leg over the knee. E. the second piece of tape encircles the leg above the ankle, tethering the first tape to the leg. The tapes are changed every few days and the foot is manipulated before each taping. The felt is used to protect the skin. F. Final appearance of strapping.

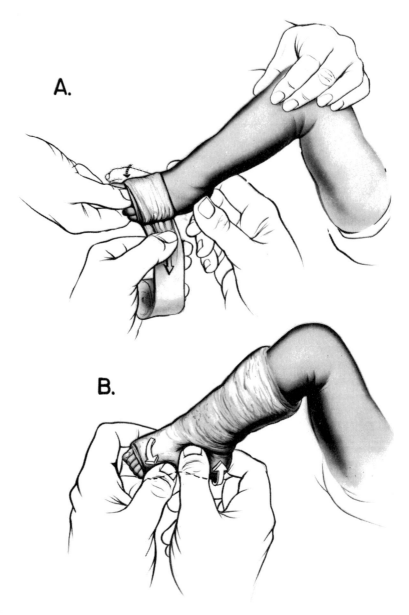

Fig. 4–3. Cast application. A. The nurse holds the toes and corrects the fore-foot adductus slightly. The surgeon applies the cotton and plaster in the direction of the arrow so as to correct adduction. The cotton and cast go on over the assistant's fingers. B. The cast is applied to the knee and the surgeon moulds the plaster with his right thumb, applying pressure to the talus and forcing the foot into abduction with the left thumb and index finger. *(continues)*

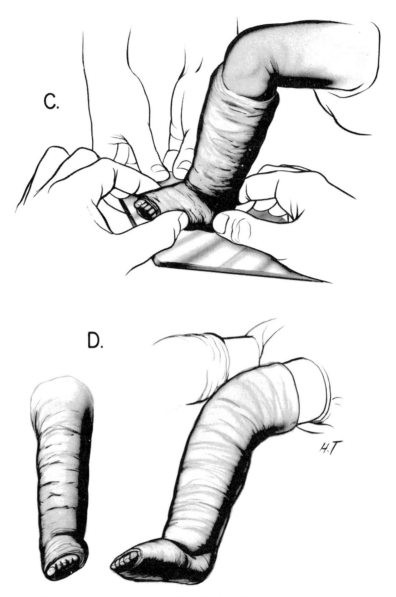

Fig. 4–3. C. The equinus is corrected by placing the foot flat on glass only after the adduction of the forefoot and inversion of the heel is corrected. D. Final appearance of the cast completed above the knee: the foot is in abduction and valgus and the heel is in eversion. Notice especially that the cast continues up to the tip of the big toe to keep the forefoot in abduction; leaving the big toe out of plaster would allow the forefoot to go into adduction.

hand, when is treating the clubfoot too late? Never! It is amazing what surprisingly good results can be attained nonsurgically in the child that is seen at several months or even 1 to 2 years of age; manipulative casts can be effective in almost all age groups, even if only a partial correction is obtained. Drs. Herold and Torok, in a later chapter in this book, show that the older child and even the neglected adult can still have an effective correction.

Before I discuss our method of nonoperative treatment, let me emphasize that forceful manipulation of the tiny foot is not without its bad effects, and one should be prepared to stop manipulations and cast corrections if it is obvious that they are not accomplishing anything. The soft cartilage of the bones of the feet can certainly be damaged by so-called gentle manipulations and also by the vigorous heavy-handed surgeon performing the procedures advocated in this volume. The point is, gentleness will give us the best result. If force is necessary, we must look again for the anatomy and mechanism of motion of the subtalar and talonavicular joints to determine what is preventing correction.

In our clinic the pediatricians and obstetricians are aware that we want to see the deformed foot early — in the first few hours after birth, if possible, although I am sure if treatment starts within 24 to 48 hours we are not losing our opportunity. The difficult foot is hard to correct, not because it was treated after 24 hours, but because it was a rigid type II or III clubfoot. The child's foot is evaluated clinically, classified as·Type I, II, or III, photographed, and x-rayed. X-rays should include an A-P and lateral of the foot and A-P and frog lateral of the pelvis. We now have a basis on which to evaluate our treatment. If the child has some underlying medical problem which might prevent us from applying a cast, manipulations are taught to the nurse or parents to use until such time as a cast can be applied (Fig. 4–1). In some areas of Europe, manipulation of the foot with strapping is done. (Fig. 4–2). In our clinic manipulative casts are used in the manner of Kite (Fig. 4–3) (Lloyd-Roberts, 1971; Shaw, 1972; Kite, 1964; Kite, 1972; Vesely, 1972).

We use soft cotton (Webril) and fast-acting gypsona plaster (Johnson & Johnson). It is most important that a nurse properly trained to assist in the application of a plaster cast be available. Holding the foot properly while the surgeon applies the cast is essential. Having the mother available to soothe the child or offer a bottle of milk is a great help. We have been painting the skin with an adherent such as tincture of benzoin and using above-knee casts with the knee in 60 degrees of flexion to prevent the casts from slipping off the child before they are ready for a change of plaster. Soft cotton is then applied to the foot and leg below the knee. The cotton is applied over the assistant's fingers as shown in Fig. 4–3 A; the assistant's right hand holds the foot between finger and thumb. The surgeon applies the cotton in a reverse direction, pulling the foot into abduction. The gypsona is then applied to the midcalf. In a right clubfoot cast, the fingers of the surgeon's left hand, mainly the first index finger, pull the heel out of inversion; the pulp of the thumb of the left hand fits in the sinus tarsi and hold the head of the talus medially. The thumb of the right hand pushes on the first metatarsal to push the foot out of adductus and also

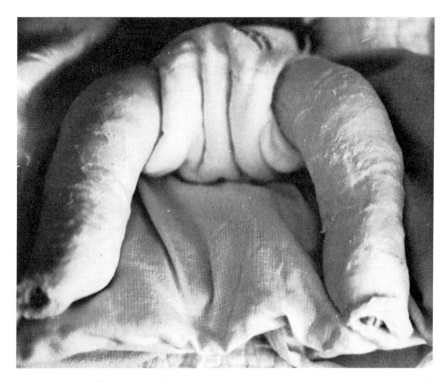

Fig. 4–4. Finished bilateral casts. Notice above the knee casts. Only as much correction as could be accomplished gently was done.

everts the forefoot. Pressure sores are prevented by applying the correct amount of padding (Webril) and not using too much force. The equinus as in Kite's method is not corrected until the calcaneus is out of varus or inversion — the calcaneus has been rotated off the talus. This may be determined by either taking an x-ray in the A-P view and observing that Kite's angle is corrected or by tickling the foot and seeing that the foot goes up and out in the everted position. This usually occurs after 6 to 12 weeks of plaster corrections done weekly or bi-weekly. The equinus is corrected by placing a flat surface (such as a glass plate or the palm of the hand) on the bottom of the foot, and after the forefoot and heel are placed out of inversion the foot is dorsiflexed. During all these procedures, care is taken to keep the heel down by holding it between the index finger and thumb of the left hand. Once the manipulations are done, the cast is completed above the knee (Fig. 4–4). If you can be sure that the cast will not slip off the foot, the above the knee part is probably not essential.

The equinus is usually corrected in 3 or 4 casts only after the inversion of the heel is corrected. If the inversion of the heel is not corrected and equinus correction is attempted, a "rocker-bottom" foot will result — the foot is appar-

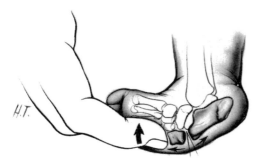

Fig. 4–5. Rocker-bottom foot resulting from forceful attempts to correct equinus before the heel is rotated off the talus—see the break in the midtarsal joint. This is very difficult to correct once it occurs.

ently corrected, however the equinus is not corrected at the heel, but in the midtarsal joint (Fig. 4–5). The casts are reapplied until the foot stays in the corrected position or assumes the corrected position when the sole of the foot is tickled.

I use a Denis Browne bar—subsequently at least until the child is walking, at first for 24 hours a day and then only for sleeping. Sometimes I even use the D-B bar after the child is walking for a period of time (Fig 4–6A). When the child begins walking an outflare shoe is worn to prevent recurrent adductus (Fig. 4–6B). I insist that the parents or physiotherapist continue an exercise program including eversion of the heel, abductus of the forefoot, and dorsiflexion of the foot, both actively and passively. These exercises are continued for at least one year.

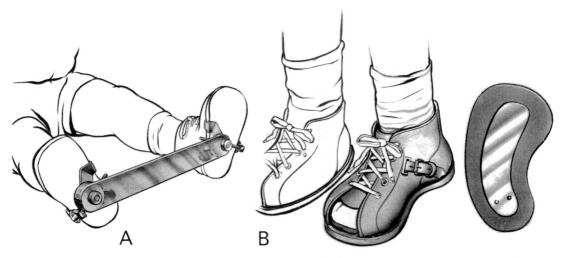

Fig. 4–6. A. Denis Browne bar, which is used to maintain position after surgery or casting. B. Outflare high top shoe for walking after clubfoot casting or clubfoot surgery. I prefer to use this type of shoe to maintain the abduction of the forefoot. The sole of the outflare shoe shows the foot turned out.

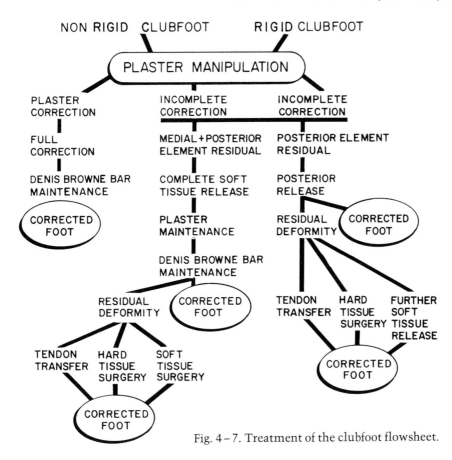

Fig. 4 – 7. Treatment of the clubfoot flowsheet.

Not infrequently, I see the beginning of a relapse during the D-B bar and corrective shoe stage – probably indicating that I have not fully everted the heel from underneath the talus – and I then go back to my plaster corrections until correction is obtained or acknowledge that surgery is inevitable. I then proceed according to the flow sheet (Fig. 4 – 7).

# REFERENCES

da Paz, Jr., A. C., and de Souza, V.: Talipus equino varus: Pathomechanical basis of treatment. Orthopedic Clinics of N. A. 9:1, 171, 1978.

Kite, J. H.: The Clubfoot. New York, London, Grune & Stratton, 1964.

Kite, J. H.: Non-operative treatment of congenital clubfoot. Clinical Orthop. 84:29, 1972.

Lloyd-Roberts, G. C.: Orthopaedics in Infancy and Childhood. London, Butterworths, 1971.

Shaw, N. E.: The early management of clubfoot. Clinical Orthop. 84:39, 1972.

Vesely, D.: A method of application of a clubfoot cast. Clinical Orthop. 84: 47, 1972.

# 5 SOFT TISSUE SURGERY

Now that the student and operating surgeon have established that the latter is faced with a rigid unyielding clubfoot, usually with a small, high-placed heel, he must make his first major decision—to stop manipulation of the foot and proceed to surgical release. The first question to ask is at what age and at what stage of the treatment we should stop conservative treatment and proceed to surgery.

Soft tissue surgery of the clubfoot is a difficult, delicate procedure and, as Turco (1971) has indicated, might be easier if the patient is operated on after 6 months to 1 year of age. Certainly the structures are easier to see the older the child is. Turco has gone so far as to suggest that if the decision to operate is reached before the child is 6 months of age, plaster correction should be continued until he is 6 months to 1 year old.

On the other hand, it is obvious that applying plaster casts early in the neonatal period is advised because of the rapidly developing growth deformities and rigid fixation contractures that occur soon after birth. If this is the case and manipulations of the foot are unsuccessful in the first few weeks of life, should we not surgically release the foot before fixed deformities and contractures occur? Is the spectacular improvement seen initially in plaster corrections false and incomplete, leading to later fixed hindfoot equinus; do inversion of the heel and adductus of the forefoot require much more extensive operative procedures (Pous and Dimeglio, 1978)? With the progress of microsurgery and pediatric surgery, Pous and Dimeglio propose neonatal clubfoot surgery, within the first 3 weeks of life. I am unable to determine at this early stage whether conservative measures have failed and, therefore, I would not consider surgery until later—at least 6 weeks to 3 months. This is when I usually make my decision for soft tissue release if I have done the initial manipulations. In those patients I do not see until later stages in their disease, I have considered soft tissue surgery from 3 months of age to adult life.

Attenborough (1972) has suggested soft tissue surgery as early as 6 to 8 weeks, however, although I agree soft tissue surgery should be considered at this stage I think, the limited posterior release is inadequate in most cases since it does not derotate the calcaneus from the talus. Concern about scar tissue contractures after soft tissue surgery making further surgical attempts more difficult is a definite argument for avoiding early soft tissue surgery, but I think scar tissue is mainly due to poor postoperative care, indelicate surgery, and improper choice of technique which doomed the foot to failure. I am very interested in hearing more concerning long-term follow-up from those surgeons who are doing neonatal clubfoot surgery (Denham, 1967; Reimann, 1974). At present, I believe indication for soft tissue surgery occurs at any age that I have given up on manipulation. Although the first time I see a child with a clubfoot I usually make a tentative decision whether or not this child will require soft tissue release, I am often very pleasantly surprised as to the amount of correction I sometimes obtain in those feet I have classified as rigid. My approach corresponds closest to Lovell's (1970), who suggests that if correction could not be obtained conservatively within a 3-month period, then operative correction should be attempted.

Once the decision has been made to perform surgery, we must decide on the necessary procedure or procedures. The operation which I will describe in detail is similar to the operations of Codivilla (1906), Bost (1960), Turco (1971), and Bethem (1978). The surgeon must be prepared, not to perform a fixed procedure as though all clubfeet were the same, but to do either as little as necessary, such as an Achilles tendon release, or as much as necessary, including posterior release, medial release, adductor release, syndesmectomy, and plantar release. The surgeon should not begin the treatment of the clubfoot unless he is prepared to undertake as little or as much of these procedures as are necessary. It would be shortsighted to hope that all clubfeet will be helped by one specific procedure, depending on what procedure the surgeon is capable of performing. I must reiterate that the clubfoot surgeon must be prepared to do all that is necessary to release the talocalcaneonavicular joint. He must also be prepared, in neonatal surgery, for very delicate surgery with very small structures, using microsurgery techniques if necessary. The knowledge of the anatomy of the clubfoot is essential. Patience and care are necessary to prevent damage to the neurovascular bundle, cartilage surfaces, and tiny structures, which should be left intact. The surgical technique required of the orthopedic surgeon in pinning a hip or reducing a fracture of the tibia has no place in clubfoot surgery.

I do the procedure sitting down with one assistant and a scrub nurse. A tourniquet is used for approximately 1 hour. It should not take more than 1 hour to do the extensive, complete one-stage, radical posteromedial release. If both feet are involved they are both done at one sitting, although we are prepared to perform different procedures if necessary for each foot. There are some surgeons who advocate doing the posteromedial release in two stages—posterior first and medial several weeks later. However, I do not believe that the subtalar joint can be corrected posteriorly and would recommend that the surgeon learn to do the procedure quickly in one stage.

## Operative Technique—Posteromedial Release

### Incision

One of the reasons given in the past for not performing the combined posteromedial procedure was the high incidence of skin breakdown. The incision most recommended was a long posteromedial incision extending several inches above the medial malleolus along the inner side of the Achilles tendon, curving below the medial malleolus to the base of the first metatarsal base. I suspect that the upper part of this incision did much to compromise the blood supply of the skin flaps. The incision we use is straight, extending from the base of the first metatarsal to the Achilles tendon under the medial malleolus (Fig. 5–1A). Since we have begun using this incision, we have had no necrosis of skin flaps. On occasions I have had to use a derotation flap, as described by Bethem (1978), if closure was difficult. This exposure is adequate for the posterior release as well as medial release, and a second incision is unnecessary.

### Procedure

It is most important that all structures are seen, especially in the small 3-month-old or younger foot. As stressed by Turco (1971) and Codivilla (1906) if the following structures are visualized and released, the entire procedure is greatly facilitated.

The following six structures have to be identified and dealt with in a special manner (Fig. 5–1B).

*1. Posterior tibial tendon.* The posterior tibial tendon is the first structure to be identified. It inserts mostly into the navicular which is usually displaced medially, and therefore the tendon sometimes has a more downward and medial appearance. The tendon sheath should be completely freed to behind and at least an inch above the ankle joint.

*2. Flexor digitorum longus tendon.* Sometimes confused with the posterior tibial tendon, the flexor digitorum longus is located just below the posterior tibial tendon and also should be freed of its tendon sheath to behind the ankle joint.

*3. Neurovascular bundle.* Just below the flexor digitorum, we find the neurovascular bundle which includes the posterior tibial vein and posterior tibial artery and nerve. This may also take a more vertical direction than

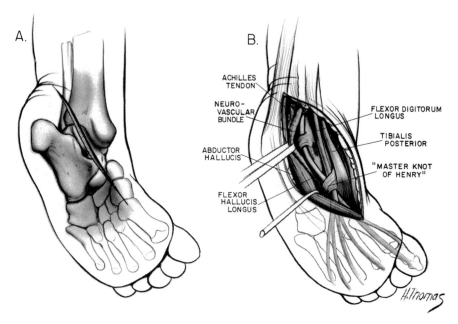

Fig. 5–1. Incision posteromedial release. A. Straight incision from the base of the first metatarsal to the Achilles tendon. B. View of the *six* important structures: (1) tibialis posterior tendon, (2) flexor digitorum longus, (3) neurovascular bundle, (4) abductor hallucis muscle and tendon, (5) flexor hallucis longus, (6) Achilles tendon.

expected. The bundle must be freed and displaced posteriorly after mobilizing the bundle behind the ankle from superior to inferior, as far as the incision will allow. It is at this point that the abductor hallucis tendon is encountered.

*4. Abductor hallucis muscle and tendon.*    Locating this rather large muscle and long tendon that insert into the tibial side of the proximal phalanx of the big toe is essential to the proper visualization of the plantar vessels and nerves. The entire muscle and tendon should be freed from calcaneus to as far as the incision will allow.

*5. Flexor hallucis longus tendon.*    After the neurovascular bundle is retracted posteriorly, the flexor hallucis can be seen to run on the posterior medial aspect of the ankle joint. It sometimes is very elusive and occasionally is seen only as the posterior release is in progress. The tendon sheath should be excised and the muscle mobilized. If difficulty is encountered in finding the flexor hallucis tendon, looking under the sustentaculum tali will isolate it.

*6. Achilles tendon.*    The lowermost portion of the Achilles tendon should be seen in the very back part of the wound. As much of the tendon sheath as possible should be excised at this stage.

I usually begin my release by considering three separate stages of release:

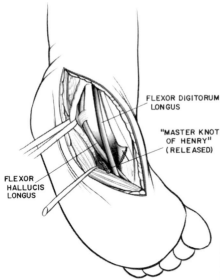

FLEXOR DIGITORUM LONGUS

"MASTER KNOT OF HENRY" (RELEASED)

FLEXOR HALLUCIS LONGUS

Fig. 5–2. "Master knot of Henry." Opening up the entire medial and posterior aspects of the release.

(1) posterior, (2) medial, (3) subtalar. In addition, I sometimes have to include a resection or release of the abductor hallucis tendon and muscle. The opening up of the entire posterior aspect of the ankle and subtalar joint is facilitated by excising the *"master knot of Henry"* (Fig. 5–2). This is a very thick heavy structure made up of fibrous tissue and cartilage which extends from the navicular around the flexor digitorum longus and flexor hallucis longus tendons to reattach to the navicular or the fascia of the flexor hallucis brevis (Henry, 1958). The knot is sometimes included in a large mass of scar tissue and cartilage which is partly attached to the navicular and medial malleolus and may be the primary tissue holding the navicular in its displaced position (Kleiger, 1962).

After identifying the six structures, I then direct my attention to the posterior aspect of the incision and start my posterior release. Let me again state that as the following structures are released the correction is tested. When I feel the calcaneus has rotated out of inversion and is out of equinus and the navicular is out of its medially displaced position, I obtain a lateral x-ray in the operating room as previously described (Fig. 1–7); if the talocalcaneal angle is no longer parallel and there is overlapping of the anterior horn of the calcaneus, the operation is over and I close.

*Posterior release.*    The structures to be released are:

1. *Achilles tendon*
2. *Posterior capsule of the ankle joint*
3. *Posterior capsule of the subtalar joint*
4. *As much of the deltoid ligament as can be easily seen*

5. *Calcaneofibular ligament.*

6. *Interosseous ligament of the subtalar joint, if it can be seen. If not, it is released during the medial release.*

7. *Tibiofibular ligament and interosseous ligament of the distal tibiofibular joint if this is preventing dorsiflexion of the talus (syndesmectomy)*

I first lengthen the Achilles tendon, using a long oblique incision, releasing the tendon's attachment to the medial aspect of the calcaneus and ending through the upper part of the tendon laterally, (Fig. 5–3A). The distance of the oblique incision is at least an inch in the infant and longer in the older child. This release usually has no effect on correction. The flexor hallucis longus tendon is then retracted medially so it will be out of the way when the capsulotomies are done. The neurovascular bundle is held out of the way with a penrose drain. The foot is dorsiflexed as much as possible and the posterior ankle joint is found as well as the posterior subtalar joint; both capsules are transected from medial to lateral (Fig. 5–3B). During this stage, part of the lateral ligament of the ankle joint—the calcaneofibular ligament and the talofibular ligament—are transected and if the interosseous ligament of the subtalar joint is seen it is transected (Fig. 5–3C). Medially the most posterior portion of the deltoid ligament may be severed. It is at this point that, if the talus is subluxed forward out of the mortise a syndesmectomy is done—the tibiofibular ligament and interosseous ligament are severed. I find this step rarely needed, although our colleagues in England perform it frequently. At this stage, Attenborough lengthens the posterior tibial and flexor digitorum longus and severs the flexor hallucis longus attaching its proximal end to the peroneus brevis tendon. He does not proceed on to the medial release. I too may stop at this stage if the heel is out of inversion, but it very rarely is and I must go on to the medial release. I do not think a posterior release is enough to derotate the calcaneus, which is an essential step in the correction of the clubfoot.

*Medial release.*    The structures to be released are:

1. *Posterior tibial tendon*
2. *Navicular*
3. *Deltoid ligament*
4. *Talonavicular ligament*
5. *Plantar fascia*
6. *Abductor hallucis*
7. *Short flexors from the calcaneus*
8. *Spring ligament*

My attention is now directed medially and I first encounter a thick mass of tissue composed of the navicular, posterior tibial tendon, the deltoid ligament, spring ligament, and talonavicular ligament. This mass of scar tissue is what is holding the navicular in its medially displaced position. The navicular must be released and relocated back onto the head of the talus. I start by cut-

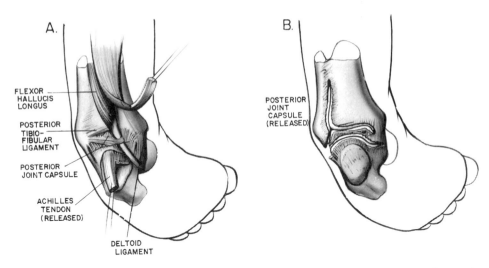

A.

FLEXOR
HALLUCIS
LONGUS

POSTERIOR
TIBIO-
FIBULAR
LIGAMENT

POSTERIOR
JOINT CAPSULE

ACHILLES
TENDON
(RELEASED)

DELTOID
LIGAMENT

B.

POSTERIOR
JOINT
CAPSULE
(RELEASED)

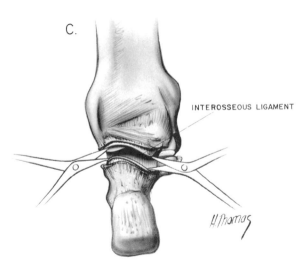

C.

INTEROSSEOUS LIGAMENT

POSTERIOR VIEW

Fig. 5–3. Posterior release. A. Achilles tendon release: method of releasing medial insertion of Achilles tendon from calcaneus and exposing posterior ankle and subtalar joints. B. Posterior release showing the released ligaments: (1) posterior capsule of ankle joint, (2) posterior capsule of subtalar joint, (3) deltoid ligament (partially), (4) calcaneofibular ligament, (5) tibiofibular ligament of ankle joint (distal tibiofibular joint). C. Posterior view of interosseous ligament of subtalar joint after joint capsule is opened.

ting the posterior tibial tendon above the ankle and using the distal portion as a handle to isolate the navicular (Fig. 5–4A). The scar tissue is excised along with all the attachments of the posterior tibial tendon to the navicular, spring ligament, and deltoid ligament. The talonavicular ligament is excised. The spring ligament is removed from its attachment to the sustentaculum (Fig. 5–4B). Every attempt is made to mobilize the navicular laterally, although this is sometimes impossible without the subtalar release which is to follow. The last step of the medial release is to free the deltoid ligament from its attachment to the calcaneus. Care should be taken at this stage to ensure that the deep portion of the deltoid ligament remains attached to the talus so that on everting the heel the talus does not evert out of the mortise (see Fig. 3–8). If

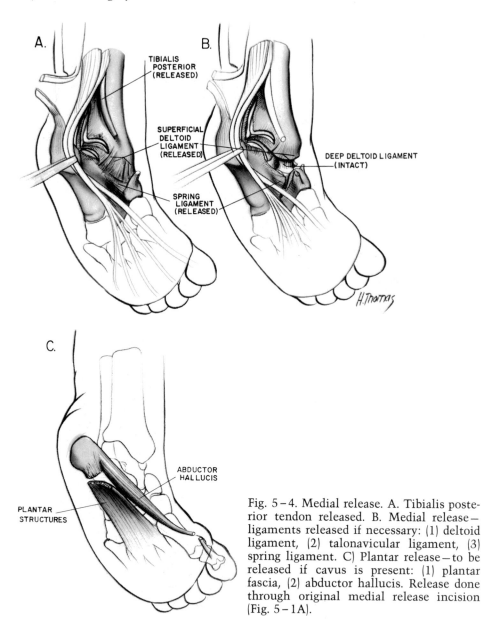

Fig. 5–4. Medial release. A. Tibialis posterior tendon released. B. Medial release—ligaments released if necessary: (1) deltoid ligament, (2) talonavicular ligament, (3) spring ligament. C) Plantar release—to be released if cavus is present: (1) plantar fascia, (2) abductor hallucis. Release done through original medial release incision (Fig. 5–1A).

cavus is present—that is, an equinus of the first metatarsal which may be present in the infant but more likely in the older child or adult—the plantar fascia is released from the calcaneus after the abductor hallucis is either removed from its insertion on the big toe or origin from the calcaneus, or the entire abductor muscle belly is excised (Fig. 5–4C). To complete the plantar release, the short flexors are released from the calcaneus either with the release of the

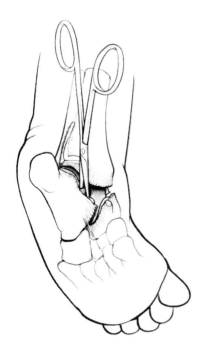

Fig. 5–5. *(Top).* Subtalar release. Release medially of: (1) capsule of subtalar joint, (2) interosseous ligament, (3) bifurcated ligament. *(Bottom).* Detailed anatomy of subtalar release.

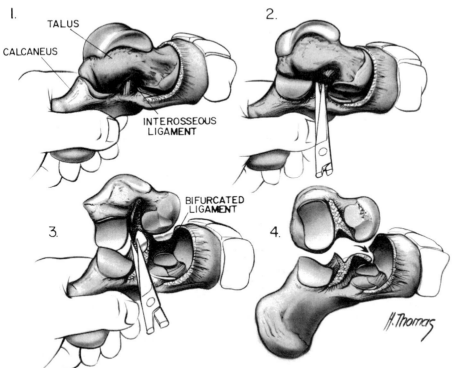

plantar fascia or by scraping the short flexors off the calcaneus with an osteotome. We now come to the final stage of the medial release — the subtalar release.

*Subtalar release.*   The structures to be released are:

1. *Interosseous ligament of the subtalar joint*
2. *Capsule of subtalar joint*
3. *Bifurcated ligament*

I evert the heel of the foot and visualize the subtalar joint (Fig 5–5 *(Top)* and *(Bottom)*). It is opened completely medially. (It has already been opened posteriorly.) If the interosseous ligament has not been cut posteriorly, it is now completely cut. If the navicular cannot be replaced on the head of the talus, the navicular must be released laterally by reaching into the subtalar joint and cutting the bifurcated ligament which extends from the calcaneus to the lateral side of the navicular and the medial side of the cuboid. It is frightening to see how much the subtalar joint opens after this part of the release and how much the calcaneus now rotates into eversion. It appears to be producing a flatfoot, but I have seen very little difficulty as a result of this wide opening of the subtalar joint. I believe the release of the subtalar joint is indispensable to the correction of some clubfeet. The last step of the medial release is to excise the tibial tendon still attached to the navicular.

The foot is now held in neutral position and, if the small toes or big toe is in the claw position due to a tight flexor digitorum longus or flexor hallucis longus, these are lengthened. The fragment of posterior tibial tendon is saved to use as a graft if needed to repair the Achilles tendon or flexor tendons.

The navicular should be reduced with care — if it is not reduced, I look back to see what structures I have not released. The navicular is then fixed in the reduced position to the head of the talus with a 0.5 mm Kirschner wire. I sometimes also fix the calcaneus to the talus with a vertical wire extending up from the sole of the foot (Fig. 5–6). All tendons are repaired. X-rays are taken before closure to be certain correction has been obtained (see Figs. 1–6, 1–7). The lateral x-ray is an invaluable guide in the operating room. Without this view showing restoration of the normal angle of the talocalcaneal joint, the operation is not finished. The skin is closed and the pins are cut so as to protrude from the skin (Figs. 5–6, 5–7, 5–8). A cast is used extending from the thigh to the toes with the foot in neutral position and the knee flexed 60 degrees.

I use intravenous antibiotics the night before surgery, during surgery, and for 48 hours after surgery. Currently, I am using cephalosporin.

The cast is changed under general anesthesia at 4 weeks and the sutures removed. If I have done only one side, I then do the other. At 6 to 8 weeks the pins are removed, usually without anesthesia.

I use casts for 4 months. A Denis Browne bar is used for night-time and outflare shoes for at least 1 year. I also teach the mother dorsiflexion and abduction exercises for the child's foot, which are to be done daily for at least 1 year.

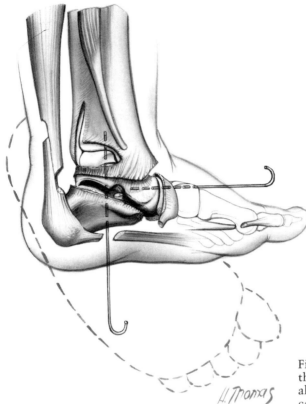

Fig. 5–6. Kirschner wire through navicular. Occasionally one is needed through calcaneus.

The results so far have been gratifying. Certainly the correction at surgery is perfect and should be unless the appropriate releases have not been done. I blame my early failures on my temerity in not performing an adequate release. However, since I have only been doing the procedure for 7 years, I cannot yet speak about long-term results.

Before I proceed to hard tissue surgery, there are two procedures that should be discussed: the very valuable soft tissue tarsometatarsal release for recurrent or persistent metatarsus varus (forefoot adductus) (Heyman et al., 1958; Kendrick et al., 1970) and the medial subtalar stabilization with posterior medial release (Schneider and Smith, 1976), which I have had no experience with but find intriguing.

The tarsometatarsal and intermetatarsal release for persistent or recurrent forefoot adductus is most valuable. I have never had to use the procedure for a pure primary forefoot adductus, and I feel as Lovell that all forefoot adductus should respond to casts. However, in a clubfoot that has persistent forefoot adductus either after serial casting or following surgery, the soft tissue release operation of transmetatarsal and intermetatarsal release has persistent and

*(Text continues on p. 58)*

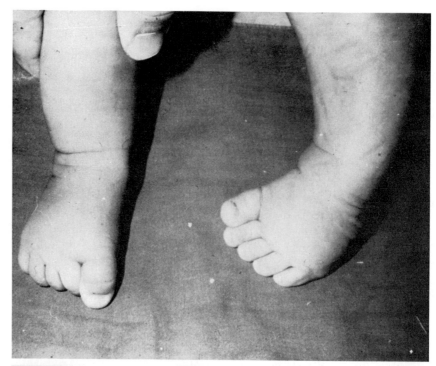

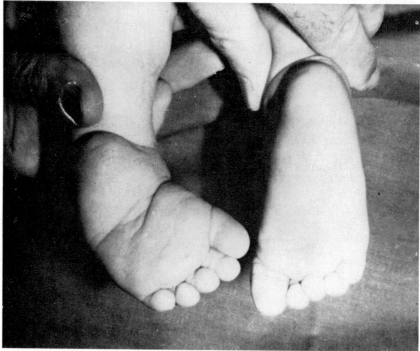

Fig. 5–7. Position of preoperative clubfoot: *(Top)* Dorsal view. *(Bottom)* View of sole of foot. Child is 4 months old. Compare size of foot with thumb and index finger of my hand.

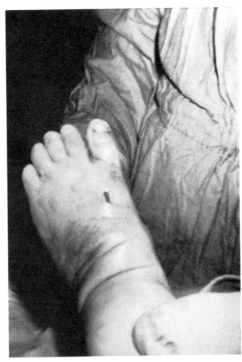

Fig. 5–8. Position of postoperative clubfoot: *(Top)* Dorsal view. *(Bottom)* Sole of foot. Note the ease of correction. No force is being used to hold foot. Note the Kirschner wire out of skin. Same patient as Fig. 5–7.

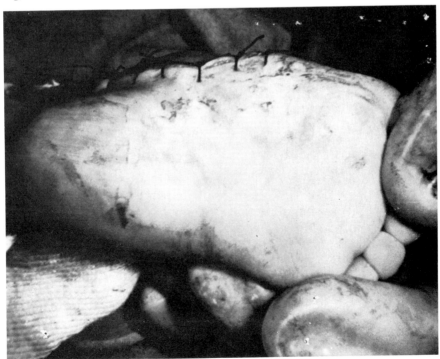

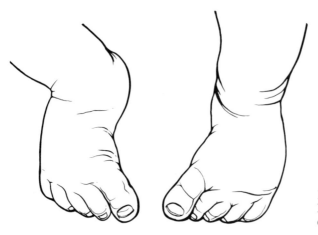

Fig. 5–9. Forefoot adductus. Patient after manipulative casts, age 2.

predictably good results (Fig. 5–9). I have very rarely had to do the procedure on patients below the age of 3 years. Over the age of 8 years, the foot is too stiff and probably only a hard tissue procedure such as metatarsal osteotomies can be effective.

The operative technique I use for adductor release follows the procedure done originally by Heyman and Herndon (1958) except for the use of a postoperative transfixion Kirschner wire incorporated in the cast to maintain the desired correction.

## Operative Technique – Adductor Release

### Incision
There are two types of incisions. The recommended incision, which is the one I use, is the transverse on the dorsum of the foot, extending from the base of the first metatarsal to the base of the fifth metatarsal. The incision is slightly curved convexly toward the toes. This is the recommended incision and the one I use. Probably just as effective, however, is the use of two straight incisions – one between the first and second metatarsals, extending slightly on both sides of the tarsometatarsal joints, and a similar straight incision over the fourth metatarsal at its base (Fig. 5–10A). However, as many as three to four straight incisions may be used.

### Procedure
It is sometimes difficult to find the tarsometatarsal space in the young child, but if you are familiar with the anatomy enough to know that the second, third, fourth and fifth tarsometatarsal joints are more proximal than the first tarsometatarsal joints, you should have no difficulty. It is necessary to sever the intermetatarsal ligaments between the bases of the first and second, second and third, third and fourth, and fourth and fifth metatarsals. The dorsal

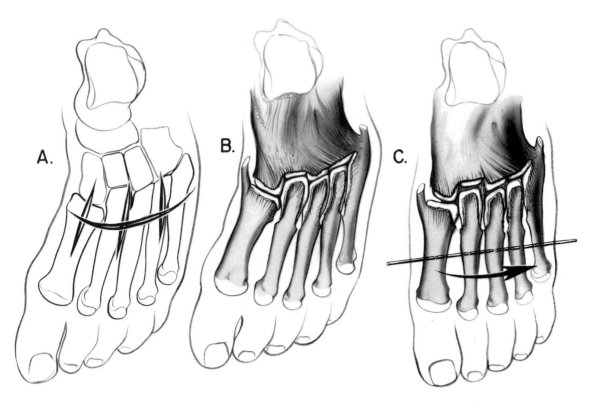

Fig. 5–10. A. Incisions for surgery of forefoot adductus. Transverse incision on dorsum of foot or intermetatarsal incisions. B. Release of forefoot adductus. Opening up tarsometatarsal joints and intermetatarsal joints. C. Release of forefoot adductus, showing final position of forefoot. Notice Kischner wire.

capsules are all severed. The tarsometatarsal joints are all opened like a book and the plantar capsule attachments are released, leaving the lateral one-third of the ligaments of each joint intact so that the joints will not become unstable. The lateral capsule of the fifth metatarsocuboid joint is also left intact to prevent instability and to use as a hinge for correction of the adductus (Fig. 5–10B).

*Closure*

I have tended to be more radical in my releases and have completely severed the plantar capsule as well as the lateral metatarsocuboid ligament. This leaves a very "floppy" forefoot, but I use a transfixion Kirschner wire of approximately 0.5 mm through the necks of the metatarsals. I leave the pin sticking 2 inches out of the foot and, using the pin as a handle, I obtain my correction and incorporate the pin in plaster (Fig. 5–10C). I use a short leg plaster for 6 weeks and then remove the pin and sutures. A cast can then be used for walking for 4 more weeks.

The procedure is effective and permanent and, I find, very valuable, though I have not yet had to use it in those patients on whom I have done a radical posteromedial release.

A deforming force very often encountered in doing a tarsometatarsal release is the abductor hallucis, which sometimes has to be released or the muscle belly completely excised. If there is an associated cavus deformity, a complete plantar release may also be done at the same stage.

One other word of advice—do not expect after doing a transmetatarsal release that the anatomy will look the same as before surgery. The metatarsal bases will now articulate with different cuneiform bones and the tarsometatarsal spaces will look different.

In pure congenital metatarsus adductus, Browne and Paton (1979) have emphasized the importance of the anomolous insertion of the posterior tibial tendon—the posterior tibial tendon inserting more into the bases of the first, second, and third metatarsals than the navicular, therefore acting as an adductor of the forefoot. In the true clubfoot, I have also found on occasion an anomolous insertion of the posteromedial tendon as described by Browne; however, in attempting a release of this tendon I have not been able to correct the metatarsus adductus of the clubfoot. I believe that the calcaneus must be derotated from the talus completely and the navicular replaced into its proper anatomical position to correct the metatarsal adductus of a clubfoot. I do not doubt that releasing an anomolous posterior tibial tendon will correct the isolated metatarsus adductus not related to a clubfoot, although I have not tried this procedure alone but usually combine the posterior tibial release with an intermetatarsal and transmetatarsal release.

I have no experience with the medial subtalar stabilization of Shneider (1976), which I find intriguing. Occasionally I have had a clubfoot deformity in a foot which is unstable because of muscle weakness, such as in postpoliomyelitis, and the child is between the ages of 4 and 10—too young for a triple arthrodesis. A soft tissue release would correct the deformity, but the foot is unstable. In such a case, I usually wait for the proper age; over 10, and proceed as with a neglected clubfoot, which will be discussed in a later chapter. In essence, this involves a radical soft tissue release followed by a triple arthrodesis. Shneider may have provided a new approach for such cases below the age of 10. He does a radical soft tissue release and then uses a Dowel graft from the iliac crest placed in the subtalar joint medially; similar to the Grice procedure laterally. I would be interested in trying this procedure in those children aged 4 to 10 with an unstable clubfoot deformity.

# REFERENCES

Attenborough, C. G.: Early posterior soft tissue release in severe congenital talipes equinovarus. Clinical Orthop. 84:71, 1972.

Bethem, D. and Weiner, D.: Radical one-stage postero-medial release for the resistant clubfoot. Clinical Orthop. 131:214, 1978.

Bost, F. C., Schottstaedt, E. R. and Larsen, L. J.: Plantar dissection. An operation to release the soft tissues in recurrent or recalcitrant talipes equinovarus. J. B. & Jt. Surg. 42:151, 1960.

Browne, R. S., Paton, D. F.: Anomolous insertion of the tibialis posterior tendon in congenital metatarsus varus. J. Bone & Joint 61-B:74, 1979.

Codivilla, A.: Sulla cura del piede equino varo congenito. Nuovo metodo di cura cruenta. Arch. Orthop. 23:245, 1906.

Denham, R. A.: Congenital talipes equinovarus. J. B. & Jt. Surg. 49-B:583, 1967.

Denham, R. A.: Early operation for severe congenital talipus equinovarus. J. B. & Jt. Surg. 59-B:116, 1977.

Henry, A.: Extensile exposure. Baltimore, Williams & Wilkins, 1958, p. 304.

Heyman, C. H., Herndon, C. H. and Strong, J. M.: Mobilization of the tarsometatarsal and intermetatarsal joints for the correction of resistant adduction of the forefoot in congenital metatarsus varus. J. B. & Jt. Surg. 40-A:299, 1958.

Hoke, M.: An operation for stabilizing paralytic feet. J. Orthop. Surg. 3:494–507, 1921.

Hsu, J. and Hoffer, M.: Posterior tendon transfer anteriorly through the interosseous membrane. Clinical Orthop. 131:202, 1978.

Kendrick, R., Sharma, N., Hassler, W., and Herndon, C.: Tarsometatarsal mobilization for resistant adduction of the forefoot of the foot. J. B. & Jt. Surg. 52-A:61, 1970.

Kleiger, B.: Significance of tibiotalar navicular complex in congenital clubfoot. J Hosp. Joint Dis. 23:158, 1962.

Lovell, W. W. and Hancock, C. I.: Treatment of congenital talipes equinovarus. Clinical Orthop. 70:79, 1970.

Pous, J. G., Dimeglio, A.: Neonatal surgery in the clubfoot. Orthopedic Clinics of N.A. 9, 1:233, 1978.

Reimann, I. and Becker-Andersen, H.: Early surgical treatment of congenital clubfoot. Clinical Orthop. 102:200, 1974.

Shneider, D. and Smith, C.: Medial subtalar stabilization with posterior medial release in the treatment of varus feet. Orthopedic Clinics of N.A. 7, 4:949, 1976.

Turco, V. J.: Surgical correction of the resistant clubfoot: one-stage posteromedial release with internal fixation. A preliminary report. J. B. & Jt. Surg. 53:477, 1971.

# 6 HARD TISSUE SURGERY

In the young child under 4 years, there is no indication to perform bone surgery. The only exception would be in a child below the age of 6 with a very resistant clubfoot, who might benefit from a lateral column shortening or a cuboid decancellation (Tachdjian, 1972). I have never done this as a primary procedure, but have occasionally combined the decancellation with radical posteromedial release when I found the foot was still resistant to abduction of the forefoot. In children below the age of 3, I have never found this necessary.

I have been satisfied with radical soft tissue surgery in children from infancy to at least 4 years of age. I have used the radical soft tissue posteromedial release as a first procedure from infancy to adulthood. As you will see in a later chapter, it is of paramount importance to use the posteromedial release even in the neglected adult clubfoot.

There are, however, indications to use bone procedures after the age of 4, either in continuation with a posteromedial release or alone.

It was noticed by Ogston (1902) and more recently by Evans (1961) that the child over the age of 3, because the dislocated navicular causes a comparative shortening of the medial site of the foot and a real lengthening of the lateral side of the foot, might do better if the lateral side of the foot was shortened. This would remove a block to the correction of the forefoot and might even prevent a recurrent deformity during growth. Others have tried other procedures to shorten the lateral column of the foot, including enucleation of the cuboid, wedge resections of the lateral side of the foot and decancellations of talus, cuboid, and calcaneus. The only procedures involving the lateral side of the foot which I use are the decancellation of the cuboid and the combined soft

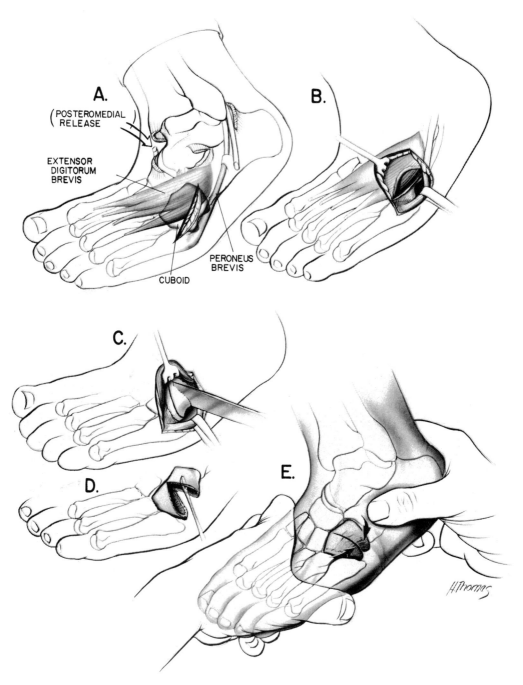

Fig. 6–1. Decancellation of the cuboid bone. A. Incision over the cuboid laterally on the foot, approximately 1½ to 2 inches long. B. Opening the fascia over the extensor digitorum brevis muscle, care being taken to avoid injury to the peroneus brevis tendon. C. Laterally based wedge taken from the cuboid. The extensor digitorum brevis is retracted downward. D. Curettage of cancellous bone from cuboid. E. Manipulation and closing of wedge to correct adduction of forefoot.

tissue release and calcaneocuboid fusion of Evans (1961). In the child under 6 who has a resistant or recurrent clubfoot, only after a radical soft tissue release I have shortened the lateral column of the foot with decancellation of the cuboid being careful not to damage the calcaneocuboid or metatarsocuboid joints (Fig. 6–1). Although the long-term results are uncertain, at surgery the foot is easier to correct after the decancellation. Although Evans recommends his procedure of soft tissue release combined with calcaneocuboid fusion in children between 4 and 9, I have only performed it in children over the age of 6. I usually start with a radical posteromedial release and if correction is difficult I proceed to the lateral side of the foot and perform the calcaneocuboid fusion. The fusion accomplishes two things: (1) the foot is easier to correct following the wedge resection, and (2) I may prevent any further lengthening of the lateral column of the foot, thereby preventing a recurrent deformity.

Abrams (1969) is so impressed with the Dillwyn Evans operation that he does this procedure in most of his clubfoot surgery; in fact, in children over the age of 2, he prefers to do nothing until the child is 4 and then use the Dillwyn Evans procedure. After the age of 9 it probably is no longer indicated. I have noticed, however, that when the Dillwyn Evans procedure has been carried out after the age of 6, the metatarsus adductus will very often need further attention in the form of an adductor soft tissue procedure or metatarsal osteotomy to correct the persistent forefoot adductus.

I have recently become acquainted with the lateral column shortening technique of lateral wedge osteotomy of the calcaneus (Lichtblau, 1978) and hope to try this technique in some cases of late (over the age of 6) persistent clubfoot deformities.

## Operative Procedure of the Dillwyn Evans Technique

I have stayed close to the technique as described by Evans with only a few modifications. The posteromedial release is done as I previously described and is not the exact technique of Evans. If necessary a plantar release is also done.

### Incision
The second incision for the calcaneocuboid fusion is over the calcaneocuboid joint, approximately 2 inches long (the same as in Fig. 6–1).

### Procedure
The peroneus brevis as it attaches to the base of the fifth metatarsal sometimes blocks the view of the calcaneocuboid joint, and therefore I sometimes have to remove its insertion. I then take a wedge on both sides of the calcaneocuboid joint with a lateral base. I close this wedge. If closing the wedge is easy, I simply use the peroneus brevis tendon to hold the reduction by reattaching it to the base of the fifth metatarsal or shortening the tendon. If the reduction is unstable, I sometimes use staples as recommended by Evans; however, it is usually not necessary after I have done the medial release and fixed the navicu-

lar to the talus with a Kirschner wire and/or used a Kirschner wire to fix the heel to the talus from below. I try to avoid the staple so it will not have to be removed later.

### Closure
Closure is routine. A plaster cast is used for 6 weeks, and then the pins are removed. If I have used staples I leave them in for from 4 to 6 months. Plaster casts are continued for 6 months. Corrective devices such as Denis Browne bars and outflare shoes are used for at least 2 years after casting.

It is not unusual for me to be presented with a patient with a persistent forefoot adductus who has already had soft tissue releases for clubfoot deformity. It is probably the most common residual deformity that the orthopedic surgeon will see. It is disturbing to the child, the parents, and especially the previous surgeon. This happens to my patients as well and cannot always be blamed on poor previous surgery or poor postoperative care. There are some clubfeet which will defy all procedures, even those done well. Forefoot adductus may also be seen as an isolated deformity not related to the clubfoot or in the most difficult of cases the "skew foot"—the foot which presents with forefoot adductus and eversion of the heel. In the skew foot, correction of the forefoot adductus will produce a severe flatfoot unless the heel is osteotomized and placed into slight varus or a triple arthrodesis is done. (See "Foot Stabilization Procedure.") At what age would tarsometatarsal releases not be effective in correcting adductus? This of course would vary with the foot, but certainly in children over the age of 8 soft tissue release of forefoot adductus would not be effective (Heyman, 1958). The procedure which is most effective in correcting the forefoot adductus is multiple metatarsal osteotomies as described by Berman (1971). His is the basic technique we use with some slight modifications. I have not used this technique in children under 8, but Berman recommends the procedure from age 6. The latest I have done the procedure is in a 17-year-old. I would think that at any age over 6 years the procedure of transmetatarsal osteotomy would be effective. The procedure may be combined with the Dwyer osteotomy for persistent varus of the heel or with a triple arthrodesis or Grice subtalar arthrodesis.

## Operative Technique of Berman

### Incision
The incision is exactly as in the soft tissue release for tarsometatarsal release. There may be a transverse incision on the dorsum of the foot or multiple longitudinal incisions (Fig. 6–2).

### Procedure
Osteotomies are done at the base of all 5 metatarsals at least ¼ cm from their bases, so as not to damage the epiphyses (Fig. 6–2B). The osteotomies may be

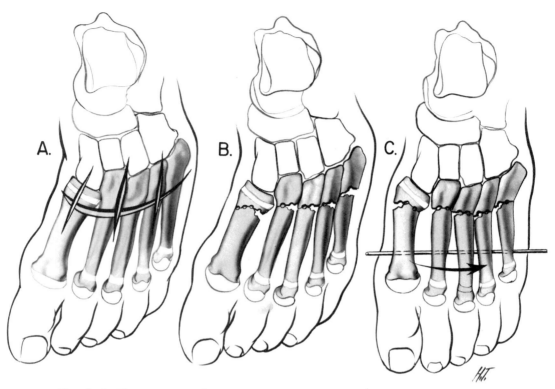

Fig. 6–2. Transmetatarsal osteotomies. A. Incisions for transmetatarsal osteotomies showing the anatomy of the epiphyseal areas. The first metatarsal has an epiphysis at its base and the second, third, fourth and fifth metatarsals at the necks. B. Position of osteotomy holes at bases of metatarsals. C. Final position after osteotomies with foot in slight abduction and Kirschner wire through necks of metatarsals.

done by combining multiple drill holes, as I have done in the past, or by using power instruments and making dome-shaped osteotomies as described by Berman (1971). He uses unthreaded Steinman pins to fix the first and fifth metatarsals threading the pins down the intramedullary shafts. I prefer to transfix the metatarsal necks with a long unthreaded Kirschner wire (Fig. 6–2 C): This wire is used as a handle to correct the deformity and then the pin is incorporated in a short leg plaster cast for 6 to 8 weeks. It is wise to have an x-ray in both the A-P and lateral views before skin closure to determine whether the proper correction has been obtained and the pins are well placed. I have found the procedure to be a most satisfying one.

The time in treatment of the clubfoot when soft tissue surgery is most effective is between 3 months and 1 year. After this period the effectiveness and long-term persistence of soft tissue release declines dramatically and bone surgery becomes necessary. However, until the child's foot has stopped growing,

interference with the growing joints of the foot is unwise. Dwyer's populariza-
tion of the osteotomy of the heel has given us a good, simple, and effective
treatment for the relapsed or uncorrected clubfoot with persistent heel varus.
The procedure he describes (Dwyer, 1959,1963) corrects the inversion of the
heel and sometimes the elevation of the heel but has no effect on the forefoot,
although Dwyer has said that in the child under 8 progressive improvement in
the forefoot may be expected with time if the varus deformity of the heel is
corrected by osteotomy. Because of the poor development of the calcaneus in
children under the age of 3, I do not recommend the procedure for this age
group. It can be performed through adulthood, but I think it is most effective in
the child between the ages of 4 and 10 with inversion of the heel. The osteotomy can be done on either side of the heel. I choose to perform the lateral closing
wedge more often because it is easier to perform. My criteria for choosing either the medial or the lateral side of the calcaneus are the following:

*Medial opening wedge osteotomy.*    This should be used with a bone
graft—if the heel is small and riding high, the opening wedge will increase the
size of the heel and bring it down. The wedge may be used in such a way as to
bring the proximal portion of the heel down (Campbell, 1971).

*Lateral closing wedge osteotomy.*    This should be used if the heel is
of normal size and not riding high. The decision whether to use autogenous
bone or "bank" bone for the medial opening wedge osteotomy depends much
on the availability of the "bank" bone. I have used the "bank" bone successfully and if it is available I prefer it. Here in Israel, Keil bone, a deproteinized calf
bone made by the Keil Company of Hamburg, is available.

## Operative Technique of Dwyer

### Incision

On the lateral side of the foot a curved incision following the course of the peroneal tendons over the midportion of the heel is used. Medially the course of
the flexor hallucis longus tendon is used below the sustentaculum tali (Figs.
6–3 and 6–4).

### Procedure

The osteotomy if done laterally follows the direction of the peroneal tendons.
An effort is made to keep the medial cortex intact to act as a hinge after closing
the wedge. A wedge is removed with a lateral base approximately ¼ cm wide. If
the osteotomy is done medially, it follows the direction of the flexor hallucis
longus tendon. The osteotomy is wedged open again, with the lateral cortex
kept intact as a hinge. The osteotomy is kept open with a graft taken either
from the upper tibia or iliac crest or "bank" bone. I have not tried the specially
shaped bone graft of Weseley and Barenfeld (1970) taken from the upper tibia,
but it certainly should be effective. It is sometimes necessary to internally fix
the osteotomies, and I think a frequent reason for loss of the graft or position of

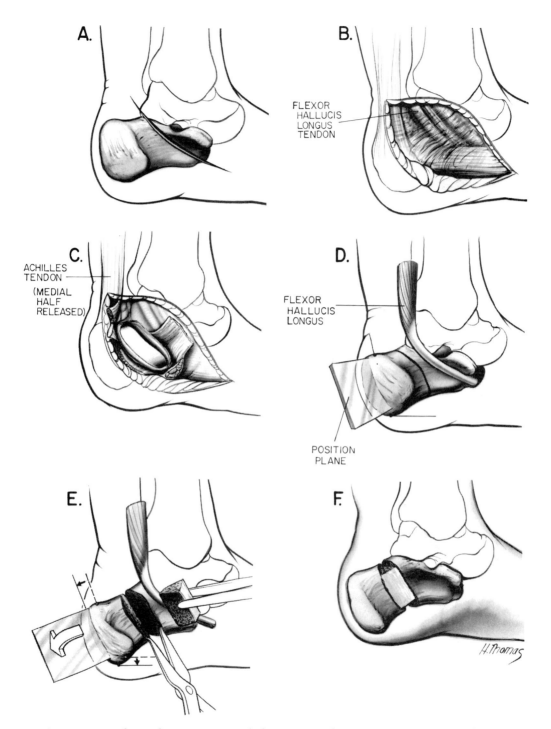

Fig. 6–3. Dwyer calcaneal osteotomy: medial opening wedge osteotomy. A. Incision for medial osteotomy of calcaneus. B. Fascia of the medial aspect of the calcaneus exposed. C. Calcaneus exposed. Notice incision releasing medial portion of Achilles tendon. D. Line of osteotomy. E. Graft placed in osteotomy site. F. Final position of osteotomy and graft.

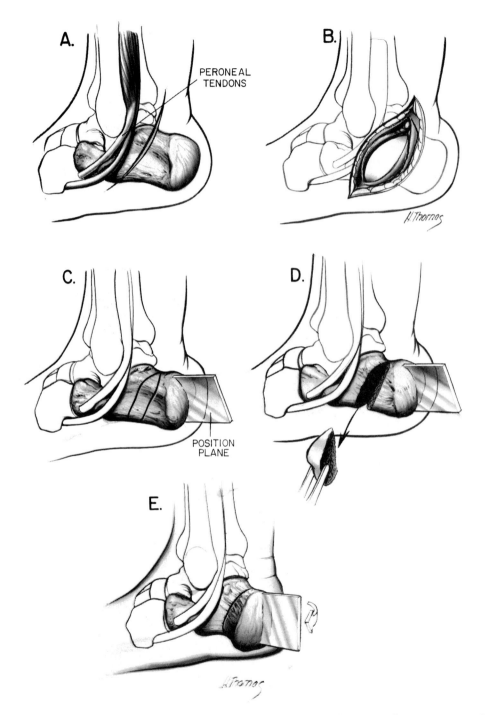

Fig. 6–4. Dwyer calcaneal osteotomy: lateral closing wedge osteotomy. A. Incision for lateral osteotomy of calcaneus. B. Calcaneus exposed. C. Outline of wedge to be removed from calcaneus. D. Lateral wedge being removed from calcaneus. E. Final position of osteotomy.

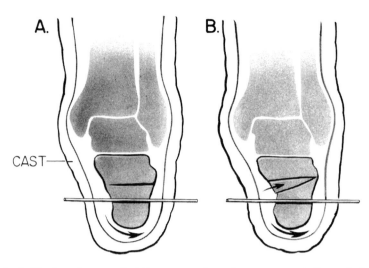

Fig. 6–5. Pin in calcaneus holding correction of osteotomy. A. Lateral closing wedge osteotomy. B. Opening wedge osteotomy. I use this method in both medial and lateral osteotomies if I need stability. A cast is used, incorporating the pin.

the osteotomy is an unwillingness to use internal fixation. I have tried internal fixation with Kirschner wires crossing the osteotomy site, but I have lately been passing a Kirschner wire transversely through the calcaneus and fixing the protruding pin in the plaster cast (Fig. 6–5). If a combined forefoot adductus procedure is necessary, I will include this at the same time.

I must add here that Dwyer feels that some amount of forefoot adductus will correct by itself after osteotomy of the heel. A plantar fasciectomy is sometimes also required. If I have done a lateral wedge I use a second incision on the plantar medial surface of the foot; if I have done a medial wedge I perform the plantar release through the same incision. I try to avoid posterior or medial releases at the same sitting to prevent compromising the skin. If I think a medial or posterior release is necessary, I try to do this first and the calcaneal osteotomy after 2 to 4 months. I also feel it is very important to release the medial insertion of the Achilles tendon into the calcaneus when doing the osteotomy. If a medial osteotomy is done, this is easy to perform; however, if a lateral wedge is being done, it is more difficult but should be done also. Part of the operation is lengthening of the Achilles tendon to take the pull away from the calcaneus.

### Closure
An ordinary loose skin closure is done. A plaster cast is used for 10 to 12 weeks; the internal fixation is removed after 6 to 8 weeks.

Much has been written about the necessity of occasionally having to per-

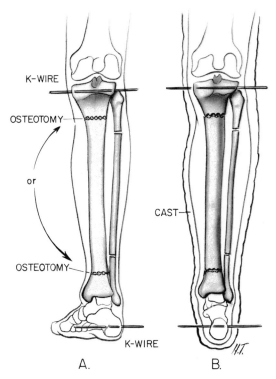

K-WIRE

OSTEOTOMY

or

CAST

OSTEOTOMY

K-WIRE

A.

B.

Fig. 6–6. Tibial osteotomy. Tibial osteotomies may be done above the ankle (supracondylar) or below the knee (high tibial). I insert the Kirschner wires first—one in the tibia below the knee and one in the calcaneus. The pins are parallel. After the osteotomy at the appropriate level, the pins are used as internal fixation in the plaster cast and as a guide to the amount of rotation desired. The fibula is osteotomized at the area preferred to allow for rotation of the tibia to occur. *(Left)* After osteotomies have been performed. *(Right)* After correction has been obtained and cast applied incorporating the wires.

form a tibial osteotomy to correct internal tibial torsion in the clubfoot. Sell (1941) has stated that even as little as 15 degrees of internal rotation of the tibia should be corrected at any age it is found and may be done is association with other procedures on the clubfoot. As I stated before, I have been unable to find any significant internal tibial torsion or external tibial torsion in the early clubfoot up to the ages of 8 to 10 (Herold and Marcovich, 1976). Nor do I think a 15 degree internal tibial torsion can be measured, especially since there probably is a very mild normal internal tibial torsion at birth which derotates during growth. However, in the adult or older child with a neglected clubfoot a certain amount of internal tibial torsion may occur, and as Dr. Torok indicates in his chapter on neglected clubfoot, for cosmetic reasons, these may have to be dealt with by performing derotation osteotomy (Fig. 6–6).

I have never seen what Lloyd-Roberts (1974) describes as external tibial torsion associated with a clubfoot, and I have never had to do an internal tibial osteotomy followed by osteotomies of the foot to bring the foot out of its subsequent adducted position. In the neglected adult clubfoot I have occasionally had to perform a supramalleolar osteotomy to correct a fixed equinus deformity of the heel. This can usually be better handled during the surgery for triple arthrodesis by taking longer wedges from the talus and calcaneus or, as recommended by Garceau (Campbell, 1971), using a Lambrinudi type of triple arthrodesis, displacing the navicular upward and thereby correcting some equinus, and at the same time performing a subtalar arthrodesis. I now prefer this procedure over the tibial osteotomy for correction of the persistent equinus in the adult foot. There is one exception, however; if the foot has had multiple operative procedures and I fear that skin closure will be a problem, I will perform the supracondylar tibial osteotomy.

## Technique of Tibial Osteotomy

Whether I perform the high tibial osteotomy below the knee for derotation purposes or the supracondylar tibial osteotomy above the ankle for correction of equinus, my technique is the same. I place two threaded Kirschner wires across the tibia, one above where I think the osteotomy should be and one below. The wires are inserted parallel to each other. The osteotomy is completed with an osteotome, using drill holes to outline the osteotomy. The amount of correction is determined by the position of the wires. These are then incorporated in the plaster cast. While doing the supracondylar osteotomy for equinus correction, an anterior wedge with an anterior base may have to be taken. Sometimes double wire fixation is not enough and a bone plate or multiple bone screws may be necessary for fixation.

Through the years we have fortunately had foot-stabilizing operations that have been used to correct all kinds of deformities of the foot. These operations described by Hoke (1911), Davis (1913), Ryerson (1923), and more recently by McCauley (1959) and Hersh (1973) have been the backbone of the late treatment (after the age of 9) of the congenital clubfoot The clubfoot surgeon has always believed if all else fails, when the child's bones are fully developed a plantigrade foot can be obtained by foot stabilization procedures—triple arthrodesis. This attitude had gone so far that Hanisch (1953) felt that after plaster manipulations in the infant the surgeon should wait until the child's bones were fully developed and a triple arthrodesis could be done. He felt that between the ages of 2 and 9 corrective shoes could be worn because he was discouraged with the failed soft tissue releases.

Today I perform the triple arthrodesis infrequently except in the neglected clubfoot and the infrequent stiff foot which has had multiple soft tissue procedures. The objective of the foot stabilization procedure is to obtain a plantigrade foot transferring the weight from the outer surface of the foot to the sole of the foot, and to change the predominant weight-bearing from the forefoot to the heel so that a relatively normal shoe can be worn. It is comforting to know there is a salvage procedure, but I think it is wrong to delay other treatment to get a normal foot at the earliest age while waiting until the child is old enough for the triple arthrodesis. Before I discuss the technique that I use for triple arthrodesis, I would like to thank Dr. Mel Jahss for teaching me the basic principles of foot stabilization procedures.

## Foot Stabilization Procedure

The basic concept is a two-plane osteotomy: one osteotomy correcting the forefoot adductus and inversion of the foot which extends through the talo-navicular and calcaneocuboid joints and the other osteotomy correcting the inversion of the heel extending through the subtalar joint (Fig. 6–7).

To better view the anatomy, I use a tourniquet with the knee flexed and the patient tilted slightly to the opposite side so that I can work on the lateral side of the foot while sitting down comfortably.

### Incision

The incision extends from just below the lateral malleolus across the sinus tarsi to the dorsum of the foot above the navicular. Sometimes more room is needed posteriorly and the incision may be curved behind the lateral malleolus. I find this extension of the incision is usually unnecessary.

### Procedure

The sural nerve and peroneal tendons are both found and mobilized and retracted. The sinus tarsi will be found just below the extensor digitorum brevis. The brevis must be removed from its attachment to the calcaneus and retracted forward to expose the subtalar joint, talonavicular joint and calcaneocuboid joint.

This is a good time to get one's bearings, to isolate the joints, and to determine what wedges of bone have to be removed. Preoperatively, I usually make cutouts of wedges which must be removed by using preoperative x-rays in the lateral and A-P views. It is most helpful to know preoperatively what amount of bone has to be removed. The sinus tarsi is cleaned of all fat and soft tissue; this step should be done slowly since all the anatomy will be exposed while the cleaning of the sinus continues. I usually take my subtalar wedge first, therefore the next step would be to open the subtalar joint; however, it is not important which wedge is taken first.

In order to open the subtalar joint, the heel has to be inverted. This is sometimes resisted by the thick calcaneofibular ligament which usually has to be cut; do not forget to repair this at closure. After the subtalar joint is opened the appropriate wedge is taken parallel to the table with its base lateral, removing the cartilage from the undersurface of the talus and the upper surface of the calcaneus. The second wedge is then taken across the talonavicular and calceneocuboid joints. I use a wide, flat osteotome which allows me to accomplish this step by taking one wedge across both joints. The direction of the wedge is perpendicular to the table with its base lateral. This corrects the adductus and inversion of the foot. Care should be taken that all cartilage surfaces of the head of the talus, navicular, superior aspect of the calcaneus, and inferior aspect of the talus are completely denuded to provide good surfaces for fusion.

The foot is now brought into proper alignment: the navicular is brought

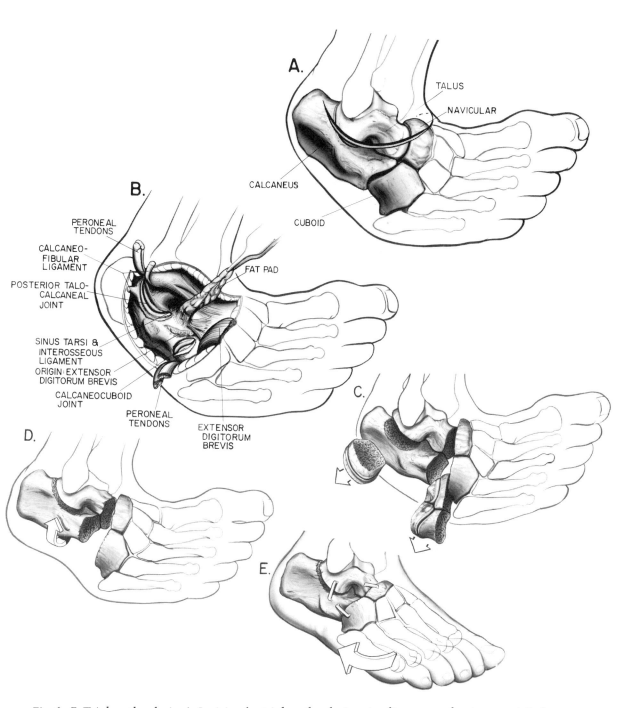

Fig. 6–7. Triple arthrodesis. A. Incision for triple arthrodesis extending across the sinus tarsi. B. Anatomy overlying the sinus tarsi. The peroneal tendons must be retracted and the extensor digitorum brevis muscle removed or retracted, and the sinus tarsi cleaned out. C. Osteotomies correcting the forefoot adductus and inversion of the forefoot, extending through the talonavicular and calcaneocuboid joints. Osteotomy of talus and calcaneus (subtalar joint) correcting inversion of the heel. D. Appearance after subtalar osteotomy. Talonavicular, calcaneocuboid and subtalar joints are completely denuded of cartilage. E. Final appearance of triple arthrodesis with staples.

lateral to the talus, correcting the adductus, and the calcaneus is brought out of inversion to the inferior aspect of the talus, correcting the inversion of the heel. The jigsaw pieces should fit if well planned, however, it is very often necessary to remodel the bone edges with a bone rongeur or wide gaps between bone contact will be found. If there are wide gaps the bone from the wedges removed may be used for bone grafts or iliac bone may be taken. I usually prepare on iliac crest preoperatively just in case. If the pieces fit and are stable — which is, unlikely — no internal fixation is necessary. I usually require three staples: one across the talonavicular joint, one across the calcaneocuboid interval, and one between the talus and calcaneus. Since I have been using the staples the incidence of nonunion seems to be much lower.

### Closure

Previously I removed the tourniquet at this stage, but because the bleeding can not be controlled I now finish the closure and cast and then release the tourniquet. The extensor brevis is reattached to the calcaneus and gives a good coverage for the fusion. The skin is closed loosely, allowing for bloody drainage which will be considerable. A long leg plaster is used with the knee in 30 to 40 degrees of flexion. I leave the foot in 5 to 10 degrees of equinus to allow the use of proper footwear. This position should be determined before the staples are inserted. The cast is split on both sides completely. Expect swelling and bleeding. I change the cast in 2 to 3 weeks to remove sutures and then reapply the same type cast for 4 to 5 months, or until I see fusion of the foot.

All clubfoot surgeons even with early treatment should have the ability to perform a good triple arthrodesis. It is a marvelous salvage procedure, but certainly does not produce a normal foot or gait pattern.

I have only infrequently had to add an ankle fusion to the triple arthrodesis (pantalar fusion), and only in the unstable muscle paralysis leg in association with a clubfoot. A true clubfoot should not need an ankle fusion.

I would like to mention a few other hard tissue procedures which may be necessary. At least on two occasions I have had to perform a naviculectomy in the adult (Robbins, 1976) in order to move the forefoot around the talus — both times in recurrent deformities following badly done, repeated soft tissue releases. On one occasion in a patient with a severely deformed foot, who had to walk on her ankle after undergoing multiple soft tissue releases, it was necessary for me to perform a talectomy (Whitman, 1901). The operation produced a very nice foot, and a much better result than I would have gotten if I had struggled with an impossible triple arthrodesis.

One case required the ultimate procedure. In a severely arthrogrypotic child who defied all our efforts and underwent multiple surgical procedures, an amputation had to be performed to allow the use of a prosthesis. In retrospect, maybe the amputation should have been done earlier and we would have avoided the multiple surgical procedures inflicted on the child.

# REFERENCES

Abrams, R. C.: Relapsed clubfoot. The early results of an evaluation of Dillwyn Evans operation. J. B. & Jt. Surg. 51-A:270, 1969.

Adelaar, R., et al.: A long term study of triple arthrodesis in children. Orthopedic Clinics of N.A. 7:895, 1976.

Berman, A. and Gaitland, J.: Metatarsal osteotomy for the correction of adduction of the forefoot of the foot in children. J. B. & Jt. Surg. 53-A: 498, 1971.

Campbell's Operative Orthopaedics. Clubfoot section, 1906–1922. St. Louis, C. V. Mosby, 1971.

Davis, G. G.: The Treatment of Hollow Foot. J. Orthop. Surg. 11:231, 1913.

Dwyer, F. C.: Osteotomy of the calcaneus for pes cavus. J. B. & Jt. Surg. 41-B:80, 1959.

Dwyer, F. C.: The treatment of relapsed clubfoot by the insertion of a wedge into the calcaneus. J. B. & Jt. Surg. 45-B, 67, 1963.

Evans, D.: Relapsed clubfoot. J. B. & Jt. Surg. 43-B: 722, 1961.

Grice, D. S.: An extra-articular arthrodesis of the subastragalar joint for correction of paralytic flat feet in children. J. B. & Jt. Surg. 34-A: 927, 1952.

Hanisch, C.: Director of Clubfoot Clinic Hospital for Joint Diseases, 1953.

Herold, H. Z. and Marcovich, C.: Tibial torsion in untreated congenital clubfoot. Acta Orthopedia Scand. 47:112, 1976.

Hersh, A. and Fuchs, L.: Treatment of the uncorrected clubfoot by triple arthrodesis. Orthopedic Clinics of N.A. 4:103, 1973.

Heyman, C. H., Herndon, C. H. and Strong, J. M.: Mobilization of the tarsometatarsal and intermetatarsal joints for the correction of resistant adduction of the forefoot in congenital metatarsus varus. J. B. & Jt. Surg. 40-A:299, 1958.

Hoke, M.: An operative plan for the correction of relapsed and untreated talipes equino varus. Am. J. Orthop. Surg. 9:379.1911.

Jahss, M.: Director of Foot Clinic Hospital for Joint Diseases, 1958 until the present.

Lichtblau, S.: Personal communications, 1978.

Lloyd-Roberts, G. C., Swann, M. and Caterall, A.: Medial rotation osteotomy for severe residual deformity in clubfoot. J. B. & Jt. Surg. 56-B:37, 1974.

McCauley, J. C.: Treatment of Clubfoot. A.A.O.S. Instructional Course Lecture. 16:93, Ann Arbor, J. W. Edwards, 1959.

Ogston, A.: A new principle of curing clubfoot in severe cases in children a few years old. Brit. Med. J. 1:1524, 1902.

Robbins, H.: Naviculectomy for congenital vertical talus. Bulletin of the Hospital for Joint Diseases. 37:77, 1976.

Robbins, H.: Present Director of the Hospital for Joint Diseases. 1978.

Ryerson, E. W.: Arthrodesing operations on the foot. J. B. & Jt. Surg. 21:453, 1923.

Sell, L. S.: Tibial torsion accompanying congenital clubfoot. J. B. & Jt. Surg. 23:561, 1941.

Tachdjian, M.: Pediatric Orthopedics. Philadelphia W. B. Saunders, 1972.

Weseley, M. and Barenfeld, P.: Calcaneal osteotomy for the treatment of cavus deformity. Bull. Hosp. Joint Dis., 31:93, 1970.

Whitman, R.: The operative treatment of paralytic talipes of the calcaneus type. Am. J. Med. Science 122:593, 1901.

# 7 TENDON TRANSFER SURGERY

What is the place for tendon surgery in the treatment of the clubfoot? All clubfoot surgeons use tendon surgery in some manner. For example, the simplest posterior release requires Achilles tendon lengthening. There is almost no surgery on the clubfoot requiring soft tissue work in which tendon surgery can be avoided—that is, the posterior tibial tendon excision of the soft tissue release or the posterior tibial tendon and flexor digitorum longus and flexor hallucis longus lengthening of the medial release. The lengthening of all these tendons is certainly an essential part of the clubfoot surgeon's armamentarium. However, when we progress from there to anterior tibial and posterior tibial tendon transfers, we encounter controversy between those like Tachdjian (1972), who do not feel transfers are of much value, and those like Gartland (1972), Garceau (1967) and Herold and Torok (1973), who believe that the tendon transfers are an essential part of the treatment of the clubfoot both early and late.

Let us first briefly discuss the tendon surgery that we are in agreement with. In doing soft tissue releases those tendons that are tight, such as the flexor hallucis longus and the flexor digitorum, especially after correcting the deformity, are always lengthened. This is part of the soft tissue release. Whether the posterior tendon should be excised or lengthened does not change the procedure or the results of the soft tissue release at all. I excise the posterior tibial tendon. In a severely adducted forefoot which I cannot correct easily during a posteromedial release, I will release the insertion of the abductor hallucis from the big toe. Herold and Torok (1973) excise the abductor hallucis routinely in their neglected clubfoot cases, and I understand Dr. Torok does this routinely in early clubfoot cases as well. If a severe cavus is part of a clubfoot, as mentioned earlier, releasing the small flexors from the calcaneus while doing a plantar release is advisable. It is after these accepted tendon procedures that we get into controversy. I will try to make it simple.

## Achilles Tendon Surgery

The "switch" operation that Stewart (1951) recommends and Turco (1971) has continued certainly has value. Stewart proposed that a good deal of inversion of the heel in the clubfoot was caused by the malinsertion of the medial and anterior portion of the Achilles tendon as it inserted into the calcaneus, and sectioning this would remove a deforming force causing inversion of the heel. Settle (1963) and Irani (1963), in dissecting specimens, also were able to show an abnormality of insertion of the Achilles tendon. I find that I can accomplish this release by removing the medial half of the Achilles tendon from the heel and then performing a sliding lengthening of the heel cord, exiting laterally from the uppermost part of the tendon. This effectively removes the pull from the medial side of the heel. I use this method in all posterior releases.

## Flexor Hallucis Longus Tendon Surgery

A warning to the clubfoot surgeon: after a posteromedial release is done and the foot is brought to a neutral position, the big toe may be found to be clawed. I usually lengthen the flexor hallucis longus at that time; however, in the very small foot I sometimes deal with I cannot reapproximate the tendon and therefore I use the excised posterior tibial tendon as a graft. I do not know if this is necessary, but the results are good.

## Anterior Tibial Tendon Surgery

The controversy is not so much over the technique as over whether (1) it is ever necessary and, (2) if it is necessary, in what cases it should be used. First let us discuss some basic principles. The foot is balanced by evertors and dorsiflexors (peroneal tendons) and invertors and plantar flexors (posterior tibial tendons). The anterior tendon, because of its attachment to the first cuneiform and base of the first metatarsal, can act as an invertor (in the clubfoot), as an evertor (in the valgus foot), and as dorsiflexor of the foot in the neutral position. It is useless to transfer a tendon and expect it to counteract a stiff foot. The foot must be placed in a relatively normal position for tendon transfers to be of any value. A transferred tendon can act to prevent recurrence by removing a deforming force or act as a tenodesis by holding an already attained correction. The transferred tendon will *not* correct a fixed deformity of the foot. In certain recurrent deformities in which a weak muscle can be seen, such as in some residual metatarsus adductus of a clubfoot with weak peroneal tendons, a transfer to replace the weak evertors and remove a deforming invertor force (posterior tibial) may be of considerable value.

I find myself doing less and less tendon transfer surgery. I have never done a posterior tibial or anterior tibial tendon transfer in which I was able to see the tendon act in a new phase of walking. The only results I have found in tendon transfer surgery are to remove a deforming force and to act as a tenodesis. Therefore, when should anterior tibial tendon transfer be done?

In the early days of medial release surgery it was felt that anterior tibial tendon transfer to the outer side of the foot was an integral part of the release. If we understand the anatomy, however, we can easily see that if the foot is corrected the anterior tibial tendon will now be acting not as an invertor, but either neutrally or as an evertor of the foot. Therefore the transfer is unnecessary. The greatest advocate of the anterior tibial tendon transfer, Garceau (1940, 1967), indicated that it was only to be done in certain special circumstances, such as proven weakness of the peroneal tendons, "bowstringing" of the anterior tibial tendon, and recurrence of all deformities of the foot. He also felt that the surgery should never be done if there is still fixed deformity. Singer and Fripp (1958) found the procedure did not increase dorsiflexion of the forefoot and relapse occurred in over 75 percent of those cases operated on. Tachdjian (1972) does not believe it should ever be done for the following reasons: (1) loss of dorsiflexion power may cause recurrent equinus of heel, (2) equinus posture of the first metatarsal may occur because of the unopposed pull of the peroneus longus tendon, (3) if varus of the foot is corrected the peroneal muscles will recover by themselves and the transferred anterior tibial tendon will simply become a deforming force acting as an evertor.

I tend to agree with Tachdjian, but since I have begun transferring the tendon to the base of the middle metatarsal rather than the fifth metatarsal I have not seen it act as a deforming force. At present I feel the only indication for this transfer is an active forefoot adductus occuring in the swing phase of gait with weak peroneal muscles.

*Technique*

The technique of Garceau is followed with a few modifications. Only two incisions are necessary (Fig. 7 – 1).

*Incisions:*  1. The first incision is made over the musculotendinous junction of the anterior tibial tendon above the ankle joint. 2. The second incision is made over the base of the second metatarsal (not over the first metatarsal as Garceau recommended).

*Procedure.*    After the first incision, the tendon is isolated. Through the second incision, the tendon is removed from the base of the first metatarsal and reimplanted into the base of the third metatarsal. I use a drillhole through the base of the third metatarsal and thread the tendon through this to the sole of the foot. I used to use a pullout suture, but now I simply use a heavy chromic suture through the tendon into the sole of the foot around a button tied over a

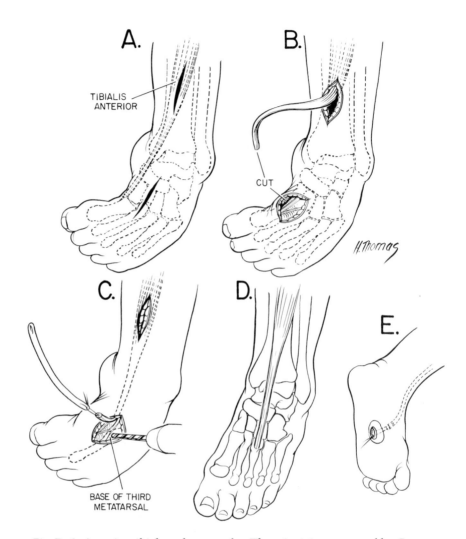

Fig. 7–1. Anterior tibial tendon transfer. Three incisions are used by Garceau: one over the musculotendinous junction of the tibialis anterior tendon above the ankle, the second over the base of the first metatarsal and the third over the base of the fourth or fifth metatarsal. A. I now use two incisions: one over the musculotendinous junction of the tibialis anterior tendon and the second over the base of the second metatarsal, through which I remove the tibialis anterior tendon from the base of the first metatarsal and reimplant the tendon into the base of the middle metatarsal. B. Releasing the tibialis anterior tendon from the first metatarsal and pulling it out above the ankle. C. Making a tract for the tendon transfer, and drilling a hole in the medial cuneiform or base of middle metatarsal to accept the transferred tendon. D. and E. Tendon transferred to prepared drill hole and attached with pullout suture or absorbable suture tied over bolster.

bolster, and either let the button fall off in the cast or cut it off when the cast is removed in 3 weeks.

*Closure.*   With the foot kept in neutral position of dorsiflexion and plantar flexion, the wounds are closed and a cast is applied below the knee. I leave the cast on for 6 to 8 weeks.

I have no experience with the split anterior tibial tendon transplant (Hoffer, 1974). I know Hoffer has used it only in spastic varus clubfoot, but it might also be effective in the congenital clubfoot by splitting the anterior tibial tendon and using its medial half to transfer laterally.

## *Posterior Tibial Tendon Surgery*

Again in posterior tibial tendon surgery we are dealing with a controversial subject. There are those like Tachdjian (1972) who do not use the transfer at all and those like Fried (1959) who believe it is an integral part of the medial and posterior release. In recent discussions with Dr. Fried I find he has lost some of his previous enthusiasm for the posterior tendon transplant because of the better techniques we are becoming used to in soft tissue releases. Certainly in the paralytic equinovarus foot with overpulling of the posterior tibial tendon the transfer is indicated, but I would wait until the child is over 4 or 5 years of age when active participation in the training of an out-of-phase muscle can occur. This may be the only indication at present for the posterior tibial tendon transfer. With our newer techniques and posterior tendon lengthening and excision of the tendon, it may not be necessary to use posterior tendon transfer at all. I do feel that in the recurrent clubfoot, whether a soft tissue release has been done or not, weakness of the outer side of the foot should be looked for and, if it is present, the posterior tibial tendon transfer considered. Be sure no fixed deformity still exists before the transfer is done. The transfer will not work against fixed deformity. Do not expect a change in tendon phase either, although it does sometimes occur.

*Technique*

The technique we use is almost exactly as described by Gartland (1972). Four incisions are necessary (Fig. 7–2).

*Incisions:*   1. The first incision is made on the medial side of the foot below the medial malleolus as in a medial release. 2. The second incision is made on the medial side of the tibia, about the level of the middle and distal thirds of the calf. 3. The third incision is made over the anterior aspect of the lower leg. 4. The fourth incision is over the third cuneiform, over the dorsum of the foot.

*Procedure.*   Through the first incision the tendon is removed from its attachments to the navicular. All attachments of the navicular on its inferior aspect are also severed (Fried, 1959). The tendon is then brought out through the second incision in the midcalf, while trying to preserve the tendon sheath.

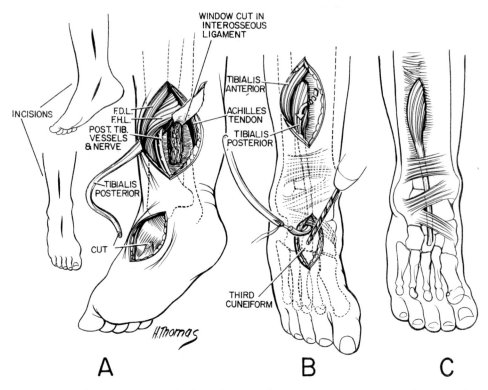

Fig. 7–2. Posterior tibial tendon transfers. A. First incision over the navicular on the medial aspect of the foot to release the tibialis posterior tendon. Second incision on the medial aspect of the tibia where the tibialis posterior tendon is pulled out. Third incision in front and above the ankle. Fourth incision over the medial cuneiform. A large window is made in the interosseus membrane through the second incision. B. Tibialis posterior tendon brought out through window and brought through tunnel to medial cuneiform or to base of middle metatarsal. C. Final position of tibialis posterior tendon transfer.

The posterior capsule of the ankle joint can then be seen and, depending on the length and freedom of the posterior tibial tendon, a window is made in the interosseous membrane above the ankle joint. A good sized hole must be made in this membrane to prevent the tendon from binding down at this point. The tendon is then passed through the interosseous membrane from posterior to anterior, brought out through the third incision on the front of the leg, and tied down through the fourth incision into the third cuneiform. At present I do not use a pullout suture, but a heavy chromic suture attached from the tendon through a drillhole in the cuneiform into a button on the sole of the foot which is tied over a bolster.

    *Closure.*   The closure is ordinary. The cast remains on for 6 to 8 weeks.

# REFERENCES

Fried, A.: Recurrent congenital clubfoot; The role of the m. tibialis posterior in etiology and treatment. J. B. & Jt. Surg. 41-A: 243, 1959.

Garceau, G. J.: Anterior tibial transposition in recurrent congenital clubfoot. J. B. & Jt. Surg. 22: 932, 1940.

Garceau, G. J. and Palmer, R. M.: Transfer of the anterior tibial tendon for recurrent clubfoot. A long term follow up. J. B. & Jt. Surg. 49-A: 207, 1967.

Gartland, J. and Surgent, R.: Posterior tibial transplant in the surgical treatment of recurrent clubfoot. Clinical Orthop. 84: 66, 1972.

Herold, H. Z, and Torok, G.: Surgical correction of neglected clubfoot in the older child and adult. J. B. & Jt. Surg. 55-A: 1385, 1973.

Hoffer, M., Reiswig, J., Garrett, A., Perry, J.: The split anterior tibial tendon transfer in the treatment of spastic varus hindfoot of childhood. Orthopedic Clinics of N. A., 5:31, 1974.

Irani, R. N. and Sherman, M. S.: The pathological anatomy of the clubfoot. J. B. & Jt. Surg. 45-A:45, 1963.

Settle, G. W.: The anatomy of congenital talipes equinovarus. J. B. & Jt. Surg. 45-A:1341, 1963.

Singer, M. and Fripp, A. T.: Tibialis anterior transfer in congenital clubfoot. J. B. & Jt. Surg. 40-B:252–255, 1958.

Stewart, S. F.: Clubfoot: Its incidence, cause and treatment. Anatomical-physiological study. J. B. & Jt. Surg. 33-A:577, 1951.

Tachdjian, M.: Pediatric Orthopedics. Philadelphia, W. B. Saunders, 1972.

Turco, V. J.: Surgical correction of the resistant clubfoot: One-stage posteromedial release with internal fixation. A preliminary report. J. B. & Jt. Surg. 53:477, 1971.

# 8 SURGICAL TREATMENT OF THE NEGLECTED CLUBFOOT

*Gabriel Torok, M. D.*

The neglected (untreated) clubfoot might not be a major orthopedic problem in developed countries, but large numbers of untreated cases still prevail in less developed populations.

The social and psychological impact of progress causes many of the affected patients in these areas to seek correction and thus eliminate a severe handicap in their socioeconomic integration. Moreover, the severe clubfoot deformity may appear in conditions that are not congenital.

To mention only one, severe spastic hemiplegia after a cerebrovascular accident might cause a deformity strikingly similar to the congenital clubfoot, with secondary changes developing rapidly after prolonged walking.

Orthopedic surgeons from many developed countries participate today in establishing orthopedic help and services in the developing countires—within the framework of World Orthopedic Concern or World Health Organization—and it is thus of some importance to gain familiarity with the problem involved in the management of this difficult entity.

## Definition

The neglected clubfoot is one with all the characteristics of this well-known deformity, but which has been aggravated by the secondary changes imposed on it by prolonged walking on the severely deformed foot. The results of prolonged walking on a deformed foot are:

1. Skin changes: The dorsolateral part of the foot becomes the main weight-bearing area. The skin here thickens till it reaches the thickness of a normal sole, with dark pigmentation. Often a large subcutaneous bursa is formed (Fig. 8 – 1A and B), which in case of breakdown gives rise to prolonged inflammation and necrotizing fistulae or to a trophic ulcer with no tendency to heal. Such an ulcer can appear also on the "dome" of the deformed foot, caused by pressure from footwear (Fig. 8 – 2A and B).

2. Stiffness: The adult neglected clubfoot shows severe limitation of movement in the midtarsal and tarsometatarsal joints. This limitation is the result primarily of the shortening of the capsuloligamentous apparatus as well as of muscular contraction and the shortening of the tendons. Surprisingly, the arthritic changes in a neglected clubfoot are generally less severe than one would anticipate in such a deformity which involves severe joint incongruity and subluxation (Fig. 8 – 3A and B). The only possible explanation for this phenomenon is that the primary malformation allows long-term adaptation. The relative absence of osteoarthritic changes was again and again proved in exploration showing cartilage-covered joint surfaces with mild erosion even in severe deformity. The exception is the clubfoot which, although neglected, at some stage underwent some attempts at correction. Here a "flat dome talus" is often found with progressive involvement of the ankle joint, and the secondary arthritis may be severe.

3. Pain: This is not a prominent symptom of the neglected clubfoot. It appears late in the forties and fifties and is seldom if ever the main indication for surgery.

## Function

The ability for prolonged, painless walking in most cases of the neglected clubfoot is generally satisfactory. Running is difficult, but many patients do not feel limited in most activities, including jumping. As a matter of fact, one should be extremely cautious in promising improvement in function after the correction of a neglected clubfoot.

## Indication

With, as previously stated, the functional limitation being relatively slight, the secondary osteoarthritis not very pronounced, and pain developing only in the later stages, the main indication for treatment is (apart from the occasional need to bring a chronic ulcer to healing) cosmetic.

This is the main motivation for most patients seeking treatment for a neglected clubfoot. It is of utmost importance to make sure that the initiative actually comes from the patient himself and not from the parents, teacher, or social worker (Fig. 8 – 4A, B, C, D, E).

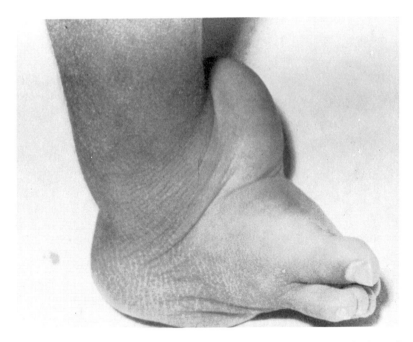

Fig. 8 – 1A. Untreated clubfoot, five-year-old boy. Note enlarged and thickened skin on outer side of foot.

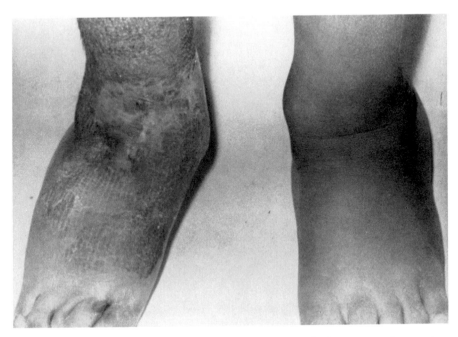

Fig. 8 – 1B. Appearance of foot after correction. Only first stage of operation was necessary.

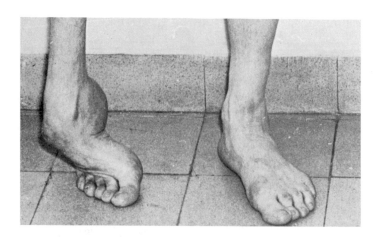

Fig. 8–2A. A 62-year-old postman had to stop work because of recurrent infections around the site of a trophic ulcer at the apex of his clubfoot.

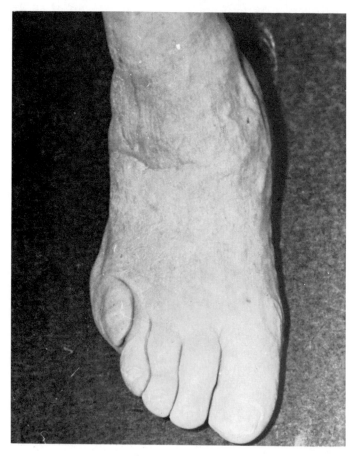

Fig. 8–2B. After successful correction he completed his term until retirement and still works in his garden.

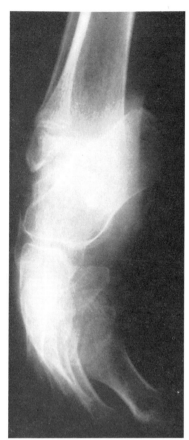

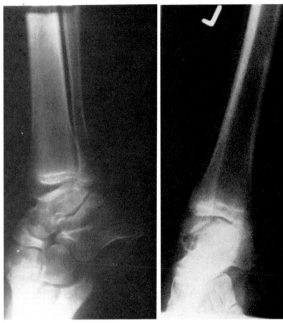

Fig. 8–3. *(Left)* A severely deformed but untreated clubfoot has surprisingly little osteoarthritic changes. *(Above)* Treated and relapsed clubfoot. Note early osteoarthritic changes: deformed tarsal scaphoid and "flat dome" talus. It is the treated and forcefully corrected foot that develops early osteoarthritic changes and "flat dome" talus.

The patient's problems should be discussed with him in detail. The involved risk, the prolonged inconvenience, and the possible pain should be explained in clear terms. After clarification, it is our custom to recommend to the prospective candidate a meeting with a patient who already finished his treatment, and then to delay decision until the patient's motivation and expectations are beyond doubt. During this process, I try to maintain a neutral attitude, as if to say: "If you really wish correction and are well aware of the difficulties, we can offer you our good services" (Fig. 8–5).

This approach spares us at the beginning, the disappointments experienced when the decision has been made on a not strongly personal basis and without due psychological preparation.

The reward for our effort in this field is the full understanding and appreciation of the achieved results by the motivated patient who evaluates properly the gain in appearance, socioeconomic status (acceptability), and self-respect.

*(Text continues on p. 95)*

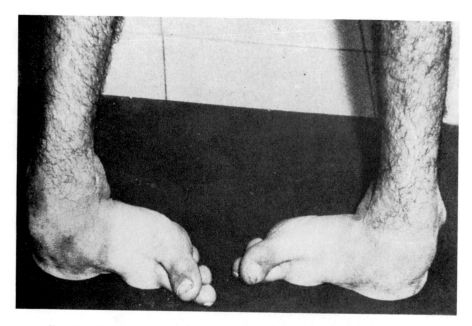

Fig. 8–4A. Neglected clubfoot. Extreme deformity in a 16-year-old boy. He was unable to adjust in society and was ready for any hardship in order to get his feet corrected. Note the similarity of the severe untreated clubfoot to the functioning hand.

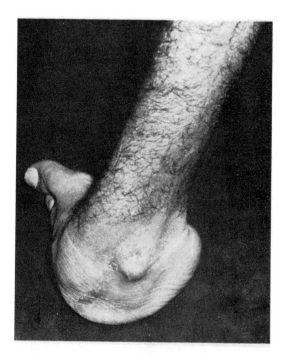

Fig. 8–4B. Side view of same foot.

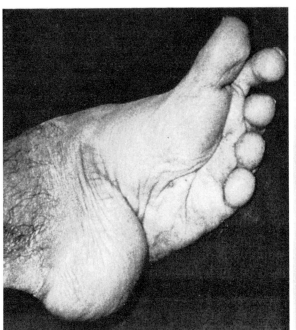
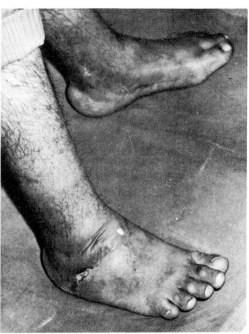

Fig. 8–4C. *(Left)* Sole of same foot.

Fig. 8–4D. *(Right)* End result after 5 years. Patient is now 30 years old, happily married, wears factory-made shoes and is fully employed as a clerk.

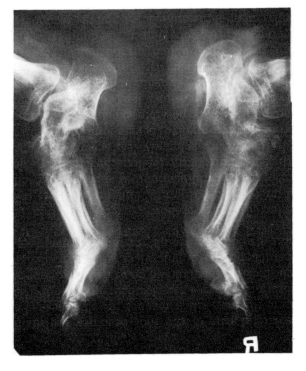

Fig. 8–4E. X-ray of same feet. Good fusion has been attained. Ankle joint good.

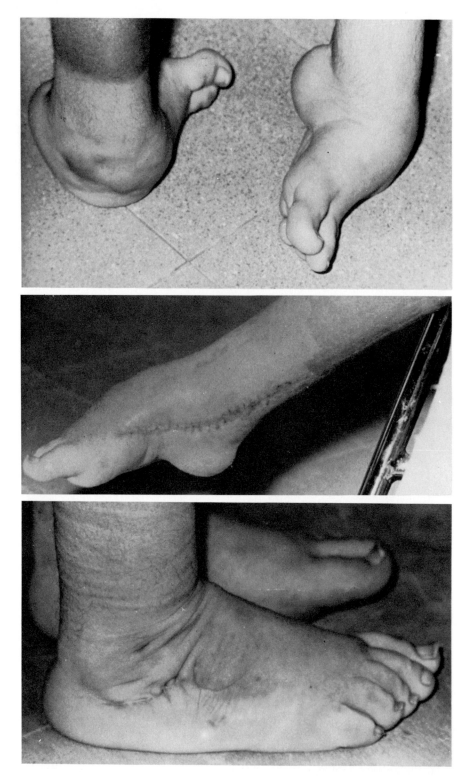

94

Fig. 8–5. *(Top)* Neglected clubfoot, 17-year-old girl. Her fiance promised to marry her if she had correction of the severely deformed feet. There can hardly be a better motivation. *(Center)* The amount of correction achieved by the soft tissue procedure only. *(Bottom)* The end result.

## Treatment

In considering the complexity of the deformity with the three primary components — equinus, varus, adduction of the forefoot — and the many possible secondary components, such as tibial torsion and metatarsal adduction, it becomes evident that it is extremely difficult to achieve all the necessary correction in one stage. It is true that the extent of required bone surgery is in direct relation to soft part shortening, not to mention neurovascular and skin problems. Thus to limit the extent of bone resection and for neurovascular safety the two-staged operative procedure was developed and adopted.

### Technique (Herold and Torok, 1973)

The first stage operation is an extensive soft tissue dissection and release. The curved posteromedial incision runs along the posteromedial border of the Achilles tendon, under the medial malleolus, along the medial border of the foot to the base of the big toe. The skin is retracted and the abductor hallucis muscle and tendon are identified. The tendon of this muscle at the base of the big toe should be detached and elevated and the whole muscle belly resected. This is an important part of the operation which aside from eliminating a deforming factor, serves two purposes: easy exposure of the neurovascular bundle and facilitation of the closure by removal of this space-occupying structure.

The crossing of the long plantar tendons is viewed together with the "master knot of Henry." Cut the knot and retract the tendons and the neurovascular bundle soleward. Release subperiosteally the short flexors and the plantar fascia. Next open all the joints on the medial aspect of the foot and resect the capsule. Include the first metatarsophalangeal, the cuneiform-metatarsal, the first cuneiform-navicular, the talonavicular, and the medial aspect of the subtalar joints. The deltoid ligament should not be completely sectioned, only the tibiocalcaneal and talonavicular fibers are divided, to prevent the increase in any preexisting compensatory valgus. The posterior tibial, flexor digitorum longus, and flexor hallucis longus tendons are next lengthened.

The Achilles tendon is lengthened by detaching its medial half from the calcaneus. This results in an outward-pulling tendon.

At this stage the correction is tested. The limits of the correction depend on the tension on the neurovascular bundle. If in doubt, the tourniquet is released and the pulse tested. The wound is closed and the correction is maintained without tension in a plaster cast. This plaster is changed after two weeks and a new one is applied with possible further correction. Serial plaster changes are performed until no more correction can be achieved.

At 4 to 6 weeks, the patient is ready for the second operation. This second operation consists of a carefully planned triple subtalar arthrodesis, preferably of the Lambrinudi type. In atypical very severe cases, a tarsal wedge osteotomy has to be performed or added.

The main aim of the two-stage procedure is to achieve maximum correction safely, and to minimize bone resection. Any injury to the neurovascular bundle can jeopardize the result, whether the injury is directly due to surgery or related to traction during surgery or poorly applied casts.

In a few cases additional operative procedures have had to be performed. These included an occasional tibial osteotomy in severe medial rotation of the leg. In some cases in which patients complained of metatarsalgia, forefoot reconstruction was necessary. Rarely, metatarsal osteotomy was necessary to overcome severe adduction of the forefoot.

The results in properly selected and adequately motivated patients have always stood up to expectations. The cosmetic improvement is dramatic. The wearing of the first factory-made shoe for the patient in this group is generally a complete compensation for the long months of suffering. Since most patients seek treatment for cosmetic reasons, the functional limitation is readily accepted. Although the objective functional evaluation of the surgically treated neglected clubfoot is far from ideal, the patients feel amply compensated by the cosmetic results and the consequent improved socioeconomic status.

The reader is referred to chapter 5 (Soft Tissue Surgery) and chapter 6 (Hard Tissue Surgery) for the illustrations of the surgical techniques used in this chapter.

# REFERENCE

Herold, H. Z., and Torok, G.: Surgical correction of neglected clubfoot in the older child and adult. J. B. & Jt. Surg. 55-A: 1385, 1973.

# 9 CONCLUSION

There remain only two things for us to consider: (1) the complications we can anticipate following clubfoot surgery and how to avoid them, if possible, and (2) how to evaluate our results.

The complications which have occurred are to be expected in any surgical procedure. The best review of the most cases has been done by Barenfeld and Weseley (1972). Table 9–1 shows the complications I have seen. The complications occurring from the nonsurgical treatment must not be overlooked. I have not had a rocker-bottom deformity since I have gone to early surgery and made certain that before I attempted to correct equinus the calcaneus had been derotated from the talus. I now use A-P view x-rays, with the foot in neutral position, before making any attempt to correct equinus. If I have not derotated the calcaneus, I will not attempt to correct equinus.

Keim (1964) has very nicely described what damage can be done to the soft bones of the foot, especially the dome of the talus, by attempting to manipulate an ungiving foot. His term, "nutcracker" treatment of the clubfoot, is exactly what we should try to avoid. Trying 30 to 40 manipulative casts on one foot before giving up is not necessary. Not only does the talus become like a "nut" being compressed between the ankle and calcaneus, but all the bones of the foot in the infant which are soft, are also undergoing a nutcracker effect. Denham's (1967) words should be remembered: "in the infant hard tissues (bone and cartilage) should be regarded as soft and the soft tissues (tendon and ligament) as hard." I have already had the femur of an infant break in my hands while trying to correct a clubfoot—the soft tissues did not give but the bone did. I am sure that, as Weseley and associates (1972) suggest, there are other

**Table 9–1.**   *Complications of the Treatment of Clubfoot*

| Nonsurgical | Surgical |
| --- | --- |
| Rocker-bottom foot | Wound infection – including pin tract infections |
| Pressure sores | Skin slough |
| Deformed talus | Overcorrection |
| Fractures | Nonunion of triple arthrodesis |

fractures occurring in the tibia and bones of the foot without my knowledge, which would show up if x-rays were taken during manipulations. I have not seen the bowing of tibia and fibula as they have. The pressure sores, of course, are the fault of the surgeon, for not protecting the skin or using force where it just will not work.

The surgical complications seem to be less of a problem than the nonsurgical complications. Wound infection sometimes occurs, though I have not experienced this. Skin sloughs used to be common, but with the straighter medial incisions this is seen infrequently. If tight closure occurs, using a rotation flap is also helpful. The pin tracts do sometimes get a little "soupy," but once they are removed the problem ends. The incidence of nonunion of triple arthrodesis has declined since I have begun using internal fixation, but it still occurs. A painless pseudarthrosis is still a good result and should not be redone if it remains painless.

The most difficult problem I have is properly evaluating my results and comparing them to others. Table 9–2 shows the method I use, however, many

**Table 9–2.**   *Method of Analyzing Results of Clubfoot Surgery*

| | Gait | X-Ray | Type of shoes worn post-op |
| --- | --- | --- | --- |
| Excellent | 1. Heel on floor<br>2. No intoeing of foot<br>3. Walking with plantigrade foot (foot flat on ground)<br>4. No limp | Normal angles<br>1. A-P view<br>2. Lateral view | Normal shoes |
| Fair | 1. Slight or moderate intoeing accompanying walking or not<br>3. Limping | Angles less than normal range | Normal shoes, but wearing them out improperly |
| Failure | 1. Walking on side of foot<br>2. Rocker-bottom foot<br>3. Limping | Abnormal angles –<br>1. Overlapping of talus and calcaneus<br>2. Parallel calcaneus and talus | Corrective shoes or inability to wear shoes |

of the children are lost to follow-up, especially if they have a good result. More attention should be given to following the patients longer. Since most of the patients are infants, it is not unusual to lose track of them when their families move. Maybe a central clubfoot registry, where all clubfoot patients are recorded no matter who is treating them, might help.

I have indicated in Table 9–3 what we have to offer children and adults with clubfoot deformities, and I hope by looking at this list, which by no means includes everything available, the surgeon will get some idea of the wide spectrum of procedures available to him. I am also quite sure that there

**Table 9–3.** *What I Have to Offer at What Age — Uncorrected or Residual Clubfoot Deformity*

| Ages | Conservative treatment, manipulation and casts | Types of surgical procedures |
|---|---|---|
| Birth — 12 wks. | | None |
| 12 wks. to 1 yr. | Always Try First From Birth to Adult | 1. Posterior release<br>2. Posteromedial release<br>3. Plantar release<br>4. Syndesmectomy |
| 1 yr. to 3 yrs. | Always Try First From Birth to Adult | 1. Posterior release<br>2. Posteromedial release<br>3. Plantar release<br>4. Syndesmectomy<br>5. Adductor release — soft tissue (Up to age 4) |
| 3 yrs. — 8 yrs. | Always Try First From Birth to Adult | 1. Evans procedure<br>2. Dwyer procedure<br>3. Tendon transfers<br>4. Lichtblau (over age 5)<br>5. Cavus osteotomies |
| 8 yrs. — 12 yrs. and above | Always Try First From Birth to Adult | All of the above may be used<br>1. Supramalleolar osteotomy tibia<br>2. Upper tibial osteotomy<br>3. Triple arthrodesis<br>4. Combined soft tissue release and triple arthrodesis (Torok)<br>5. Talectomy<br>6. Naviculectomy<br>7. Amputation (possibly in severe arthrogryposis) |

are other ways to accomplish the same results I accomplish, but these procedures are what I am familiar and happy with, until I try something else.

As Waisbrod has stated (1973), the latest reviews of clubfoot treatment, both conservative and surgical, have indicated that only 50 percent of cases are successful. Lloyd-Roberts (1964) stated, "This is an undeniably disheartening state of affairs which is in no way redeemed by the knowledge that little or no improvement has occurred since Brockman's review was published 35 years ago" (Brockman, 1930). And he added: "What are the features that are likely to make a clubfoot resist treatment?"

It has been the purpose of this book to try to answer Lloyd-Roberts' question, and I hope that with better understanding of the pathoanatomy of the clubfoot and better awareness of the enormous variety of procedures available to the treating physician, he will be able to manage the infinite variety of stages of clubfoot presented to him. Probably no two clubfeet are exactly the same, and each clubfoot must be attacked not with simply one procedure in mind, but with the knowledge of all that is available.

This book has tried to put together in one volume what is available to the physician for the treatment of the clubfoot and at what stage it is appropriate. I hope in some small way I have helped the beginning clubfoot surgeon get things together. I have borrowed from many sources and have tried to give them appropriate recognition though I may have forgotten some.

I ask all surgeons treating the clubfoot deformity to follow their cases, record the end result, and honestly share this knowledge with us. Our only way to improve the overall results is to know which procedures work and which do not.

# REFERENCES

Barenfeld, P. and Weseley, M.: Surgical treatment of the clubfoot. Clinical Orthop. 84: 79, 1972.

Brockman, E. P.: Congenital Clubfoot. New York, Wood, 1930.

Denham, R. A.: Congenital talipes equinovarus. J. B. & Jt. Surg. 49-B: 583, 1967.

Keim, H. A., Ritchie, G. W.: "Nut-cracker" treatment of clubfoot. J.A.M.A. 189: 613, 1964.

Lloyd-Roberts, G. C.: Congenital clubfoot. J. B. &Jt. Surg. 46-B: 369, 1964.

Waisbrod, H.: Congenital clubfoot: An anatomical study. J. B. & Jt. Surg. 55-B: 796, 1973.

Weseley, M., Barenfeld, P., Barret, N.: Complications of the treatment of clubfoot. Clinical Orthop. 84:93, 1972.

# INDEX

Numerals in italics indicate a figure, and those followed by "t" indicate a table.